Epigenetics and Human Longevity

A short introduction by The HealthSpan Institute

Epigenetics and Human Longevity:
A Short Inroduction

ISBN: 9798866070077

Printed in the United States of America

Contents

Preface

Introduction to the Field of Epigenetics 15

What is Epigenetics? 15

Key Epigenetic Mechanisms 15

The Significance of Epigenetics 16

Epigenetics and the Environment 16

A New Frontier in Biology 17

In Conclusion 17

The Relationship Between Genetics, Epigenetics, and Longevity 17

Genetics: Our Biological Blueprint 18

Epigenetics: The Dynamic Layer 18

The Interplay: Genetics, Epigenetics, and Aging 18

Influencing Longevity: Is It All Predestined? 19

Future Prospects: Can We "Edit" Longevity? 19

In Conclusion 20

Chapter 1:
Basics of Epigenetics

Definition and History of Epigenetics 21

Defining Epigenetics 21

The Origins of Epigenetics 21

The Molecular Era 22

The Contemporary Understanding 22

Epigenetics Beyond Humans 23

Challenges and Evolving Definitions 23

In Conclusion 23

Key Concepts: DNA Methylation, Histone Modification, and Non-Coding RNA............24

DNA Methylation: The Molecular "Off Switch".............24

Histone Modification: The Dynamic Sculptors of Chromatin 24

Non-Coding RNA: Silent Sequences with Loud Impacts 25

Bringing It All Together.............26

The Dynamic Nature of the Epigenome.............26

Epigenetic Plasticity: A Double-Edged Sword.............26

Influences Shaping the Epigenome 27

Memory of the Epigenome: Transgenerational Epigenetic Inheritance 28

Epigenetic Resets.............28

Concluding Thoughts.............29

Chapter 2:
The Epigenetic Clock

Introduction to the Concept of Biological vs. Chronological Age.............30

Chronological Age: The Inevitable Passage of Time.............30

Biological Age: A Reflection of Internal Wear and Tear........30

Why the Distinction Matters 31

The Epigenetic Connection.............31

Concluding Thoughts.............32

The Science Behind DNA Methylation as a Predictor of Age.............32

DNA Methylation: A Brief Overview 33

Methylation Patterns and Aging.............33

Development of the Epigenetic Clock 33

Beyond Chronological Age: Indications of Biological Aging 34

Mechanisms: Why Does DNA Methylation Change with Age?.............34

Concluding Thoughts..35

Implications for Health and Lifespan Predictions........35

Health Indicators and the Epigenetic Clock...........................35

Predicting Lifespan: Beyond Just Age.....................................36

Personalized Medicine and the Promise of Early
Interventions 36

Potential Modifiers of the Epigenetic Clock...........................36

Ethical Considerations: The Double-Edged Sword 37

Concluding Thoughts..37

Chapter 3:
Lifestyle and the Epigenome

Diet and its Impact on DNA Methylation Patterns.......38

The Dynamic Interplay: Nutrients and DNA Methylation ...38

Specific Foods and their Epigenetic Impact............................39

Diet-Induced Methylation Changes: Health Implications...39

The Lifelong Influence of Early Diet 40

Personalized Nutrition: Tailoring Diet for the
Epigenome 40

Concluding Thoughts..40

Exercise and Epigenetic Age Reversal 41

Physical Activity: A Catalyst for Epigenetic Change.............41

The Epigenetic Clock and Exercise: Turning Back Time? 41

How Exercise Might Reset the Clock 42

Exercise Intensity, Duration, and Type: Finding the
Sweet Spot..42

Health Implications: Beyond Just Feeling Younger 43

Concluding Thoughts..43

**The Epigenetic Consequences of Smoking,
Alcohol, and Stress 44**

Smoking: A Cloud of Epigenetic Alterations 44

Alcohol: Beyond the Buzz to the Epigenome 45

Stress: Silent Cellular Strains..................................45

Interplay and Cumulative Effects...........................46

Concluding Thoughts..46

Other Environmental Factors Influencing the Epigenome 46

Air Pollution: Beyond Breathing Difficulties 47

Early-Life Exposures: Imprints that Last 47

Pesticides, Plastics, and Chemicals: The Invisible Threats...48

Infections and the Immune Response 48

Light and Circadian Rhythms: The Biological Clock's Influence 48

Epigenetic Memory and Transgenerational Effects 49

Concluding Thoughts..49

Chapter 4:
Caloric Restriction and Epigenetic Longevity

Overview of Caloric Restriction Studies Across Species...50

Yeast: Simplicity Lends Clarity................................50

Worms and Flies: Small Organisms, Big Insights..................51

Mammalian Models: Rodents Lead the Way.............51

Non-human Primates: Closer to Home 51

Humans: Gleaning Insights from Limited Data 52

Evolutionary Conservation: A Common Thread................52

Concluding Thoughts..53

Molecular Mechanisms Linking Restriction with Lifespan Extension 53

Insulin/IGF-1 Signaling: A Central Longevity Pathway........53

mTOR: Sensing Nutrients and Orchestrating Growth 54

Sirtuins: The Epigenetic Guardians of Longevity.................54

AMPK: The Cellular Energy Sensor.........................54

Enhanced Autophagy: Cellular Recycling at Its Best............55

Enhanced Stress Resistance: Preparing for the Tough Times 55

Concluding Thoughts 56

Implications for Human Diet and Longevity 56

Translating Animal Data to Human Longevity 56

Epigenetics: Bridging Diet and Lifespan in Humans 57

Practical Implications: Adapting CR for Human Lifestyles 57

Social and Psychological Dimensions 58

Potential Risks and Considerations 58

Concluding Thoughts 59

Chapter 5:
Histones and Aging

Basics of Histone Modifications 60

The Structure and Role of Histones 60

Types of Histone Modifications 60

Enzymes Mediating Histone Modifications 61

Histone Modifications and Gene Regulation 61

Implications for Cellular Memory and Identity 62

Concluding Thoughts 62

The Role of Histones in Gene Expression 63

The Fundamental Unit: The Nucleosome 63

Chromatin Remodeling and Accessibility 63

The Epigenetic Language of Histone Modifications 64

Histone Modifiers and Readers 64

Histones and Aging: A Dynamic Interplay 65

Concluding Reflections 65

How Aging Influences and Is Influenced by Histone Modifications 65

Global Loss of Histone Proteins and Modifications 66

Changes in Specific Histone Modifications 66

The Role of Sirtuins: From Histones to Aging 66

Histone Modifications and DNA Damage Response 67

Changes in Histone Variants with Age 67

Histone Modifications in Age-related Diseases 68

Concluding Insights 68

Chapter 6:
Transgenerational Epigenetic Inheritance

The Debate over Inheritance of Acquired Traits 69

Jean-Baptiste Lamarck and the Legacy of Lamarckism.......69

Modern Epigenetics and the Revival of
Lamarckian Ideas 70

Experimental Evidence and Notable Cases...........................70

Skepticism and Challenges 70

Implications for Evolutionary Biology 71

Conclusion: An Evolving Understanding...............................71

**Studies Supporting Epigenetic Inheritance
Across Generations**........................72

The Agouti Mouse: A Colorful Tale of Epigenetics................72

Vinclozolin and Reproductive Changes in Rats.....................72

Honeybees: A Story of Nutrition and Destiny 73

The Swedish Overkalix Study: Famine's Echo Across
Generations........................73

Caenorhabditis elegans and Small RNAs 74

Contemplations and Considerations 74

Conclusion: A Dynamic Field with Growing Evidence 74

Implications for Familial Health and Longevity..........75

The Shadow of Ancestral Environments................................75

Beyond Genetic Counseling: Epigenetic Counseling?.........75

Health Interventions: A Multi-Generational Perspective 76

Psychological and Societal Implications 76

Ethical Considerations 77

The Evolutionary Perspective: Adapting Across
Generations...77

Conclusion: A New Frontier in Family Health and
Longevity...77

Chapter 7:
Epigenetics and Age-Related Diseases

Overview of Common Age-Related Diseases 79

Cardiovascular Diseases (CVDs) 79

Alzheimer's Disease and Other Dementias 80

Osteoporosis 80

Type 2 Diabetes Mellitus (T2DM) 80

Age-Related Macular Degeneration (AMD) 81

Parkinson's Disease..81

Rheumatoid Arthritis 81

Conclusion: A Complex Interplay Between Age and
Disease 82

**The Role of Epigenetic Changes in Disease Onset
and Progression**..82

How Epigenetic Changes Occur 82

Epigenetic Changes in Cancer 83

Cardiovascular Diseases and Epigenetics 83

Neurodegenerative Diseases.....................................83

Diabetes Mellitus 84

Autoimmune Disorders 84

Epigenetics and Disease Progression 84

Epigenetic Markers as Diagnostic Tools 85

Therapeutic Implications...85

Conclusion: A Deeper Understanding of Disease.........85

Potential for Epigenetic Therapies........................85

Epigenetic Dysregulation and Disease 86

Current Epigenetic Therapies in Use 86

Potential Applications of Epigenetic Therapies 87

Rejuvenation and Age Reversal 87

Challenges in Epigenetic Therapies 88

Future Directions 88

Conclusion: A New Horizon in Medicine.......................88

Chapter 8:
Reversing the Clock –
The Future of Epigenetic Therapies

Current State of Research on Epigenetic Rejuvenation..................................90

Epigenetic Clocks and Their Significance 90

Key Breakthroughs in Epigenetic Rejuvenation 91

Challenges in Translating Research to Therapies.................91

The Road Ahead: Next Steps in Epigenetic Rejuvenation...92

Conclusion: The Dawn of a New Era 92

The Potential and Challenges of Age-Reversal Therapies..................................92

The Lure of Age-Reversal................................93

The Potential of Age-Reversal Therapies.......................93

Challenges in Age-Reversal Therapies.........................94

The Way Forward 95

Conclusion: The Horizon of Age-Reversal 95

Ethical Considerations 95

The Inequity of Access 95

The Implications for Population and Resources 96

The Challenge of Longevity 96

Redistribution of Life's Milestones..........................96

The Nature of Medical Treatment 97

Consent and Autonomy 97

The Morality of Playing with Time 97

Conclusion: Navigating the Ethical Maze 98

Chapter 9:
Epigenetic Drugs and Longevity

Introduction to Drugs Targeting the Epigenome 99

The Logic of Epigenetic Drugs.....................................99

Classes of Epigenetic Drugs 100

The Success Story: Epigenetic Drugs in Oncology 100

Broad Spectrum vs. Specific Targeting 101

Looking Ahead: The Potential for Longevity 101

Current Applications in Cancer and Other Diseases 101

Epigenetic Drugs in Oncology....................................102

Epigenetic Drugs in Neurological Diseases 102

Epigenetic Drugs in Autoimmune Diseases...................103

Epigenetic Drugs in Cardiovascular Diseases.................103

Challenges and Considerations................................104

Concluding Thoughts 104

The Potential for Lifespan Extension through Pharmacology 104

Molecular Targets of Aging 105

Pharmacological Interventions Targeting Aging Pathways 105

Translating Findings to Human Longevity....................106

Ethical Considerations 106

Concluding Thoughts..107

Chapter 10:
Challenges and Frontiers in Epigenetic Longevity Research

The Complexity of the Epigenome and its Implications 108

Epigenome: A Dynamic Landscape 108

Implications for Disease and Aging...............................109

Challenges in Deciphering the Epigenome 109

Opportunities in Epigenetic Interventions 110

Looking Forward: Future of Epigenetic Longevity Research...110

Differentiating Between Causation and Correlation in Research 111

What is Correlation? 111

What is Causation?...111

Challenges in Distinguishing Correlation from Causation..112

Why it Matters in Epigenetic Longevity Research 112

Strategies to Determine Causation 113

Caveats and Considerations...113

The Future Trajectory of Epigenetics and Longevity Studies 114

Expanding the Scope of Research 114

Technological Advancements...114

Breakthroughs in Interventions 115

Ethical and Societal Implications 115

Potential Challenges 116

Collaboration and Open Science 116

Conclusion

Summarizing Key Insights from the Book 118

The Multifaceted Epigenome 118

A Biological Clock Within...................................118

Lifestyle's Mark on the Epigenome........................119

Starvation's Silver Lining 119

The Histone-Gene Tango 119

Heredity Beyond Genes 120

Decoding Disease through Epigenetics 120

Future Horizons in Epigenetic Therapies.................120

Drugs Targeting the Epigenome 120

The Research Road Ahead 121

The Holistic Approach to Understanding and Influencing Human Aging through Epigenetics 121

The Intersection of Genes, Environment, and Lifestyle.......122

An Integrated Approach to Aging 122

Embracing Complexity and Interconnectedness...................122

Proactive and Preventative Interventions 123

Cultivating a Holistic Lifestyle 123

Embracing the Bigger Picture..............................124

Hope and Potential for Future Breakthroughs 124

From Understanding to Intervention........................124

The Advent of Precision Medicine 125

Rejuvenation and Age Reversal 125

Cross-disciplinary Synergies................................126

An Ethical Compass for the Journey Ahead 126

A Hopeful Horizon 126

Appendix A:
Glossary of Terms

A 128

B 128

C 128

D 128

E 129

H 129

L 129

M 129

P 129

R 130

S 130

T 130

U 130

Appendix B:
Resources for Further Reading

Books 131

Research Journals and Articles 132

Websites and Online Platforms 132

Podcasts and Webinars 133

Organizations and Institutes 133

Preface

Introduction to the Field of Epigenetics

In the intricate world of biology, the term "genetics" often conjures images of DNA double helices and sequences of nucleotides determining our physical and biological attributes. Yet, our understanding of biology underwent a profound expansion with the emergence of epigenetics, a discipline that explores the layers of complexity beyond the DNA sequence.

What is Epigenetics?

At its core, epigenetics examines modifications on the genetic material or associated proteins that influence gene activity without changing the underlying DNA sequence. The term "epigenetics" is derived from the Greek prefix "epi-", meaning "over, outside of, around." Thus, epigenetics revolves around changes "on top of" or "in addition to" genetics.

In simpler terms, while our DNA sequence (our genome) provides the basic script, epigenetics provides the annotations, editing, and instructions on when, where, and how this script should be read. These epigenetic modifications are like switches that can turn genes on or off, ensuring that only necessary genes are active in a particular cell at a given time.

Key Epigenetic Mechanisms

Several mechanisms underpin epigenetic regulation:

1. **DNA Methylation:** This involves the addition of a methyl group to a cytosine base in the DNA, typically leading to gene silencing. DNA methylation patterns play a pivotal role in processes like embryonic development, X-chromosome inactivation, and genomic imprinting.

2. **Histone Modifications:** DNA is wrapped around proteins called histones. Chemical modifications to these histones can affect the structure of the DNA, either allowing or restricting access to the underlying genes, thus influencing their activity.

3. **Non-Coding RNA:** These are RNA molecules that don't code for proteins but can influence gene expression and other cellular processes.

The Significance of Epigenetics

Epigenetic changes are pivotal for normal growth and development. They help differentiate the myriad of cell types in our bodies—from skin cells to neurons—even though all these cells share the same DNA sequence. The difference in cell function and identity is largely driven by the varied patterns of gene expression orchestrated by epigenetics.

However, while epigenetic modifications are essential for our physiology, they can sometimes go awry. Disruptions in normal epigenetic processes can lead to a plethora of conditions and diseases, including cancers, neurological disorders, and developmental abnormalities. Recognizing these aberrations is crucial for diagnostics, prognostics, and even therapeutic interventions.

Epigenetics and the Environment

One of the most tantalizing aspects of epigenetics is how it interfaces with our environment. Unlike our static DNA sequence, the epigenome is dynamic. It can be influenced by external factors such as diet, stress, toxins, and even experiences. This means that lifestyle and environmental exposures can bring about lasting changes in gene expression, contributing to health outcomes, both positive and negative.

For instance, prenatal exposures to certain toxins can lead to epigenetic changes in the developing fetus, predisposing them to health issues later in life. Similarly, trauma experienced during crucial developmental stages can embed itself in the epigenome, leading to long-term health and psychological impacts.

A New Frontier in Biology

The field of epigenetics has opened up vast new horizons for biological research. It has redefined our understanding of genetics, heredity, and gene-environment interactions. Instead of being passive blueprints, our genomes are now understood as dynamic entities, constantly interacting with and being reshaped by the environment.

Moreover, epigenetics also offers a fresh perspective on evolution. While traditional genetic changes (mutations) play a fundamental role in evolution, epigenetic changes provide a mechanism for organisms to adapt rapidly to new environments within a single generation. These epigenetic adaptations can sometimes be passed on to subsequent generations, adding another layer to the intricate dance of evolution.

In Conclusion

Epigenetics serves as a reminder of the beautiful complexity of life. It bridges the gap between our genes and the environment, demonstrating that we are not just products of our DNA, but also of our experiences and choices. As we continue to unravel the mysteries of the epigenome, we stand to gain profound insights into health, disease, development, and the very essence of what it means to be human.

The Relationship Between Genetics, Epigenetics, and Longevity

Longevity, or the duration of an individual's life, has captivated human interest for centuries. The quest for a longer, healthier life is a universal aspiration. But what determines how long we live? While the environment, lifestyle, and chance all play roles, our biology, specifically the domains of genetics and epigenetics, profoundly influences longevity.

Genetics: Our Biological Blueprint

Genetics revolves around the study of genes — sequences of DNA that carry instructions for making proteins, the workhorses of our cells. Our genetic makeup, or genome, is essentially the blueprint that directs many aspects of our biology, from eye color to certain predispositions to diseases.

When discussing longevity, certain genes have been identified that seem to influence lifespan. For instance, some genetic mutations can cause premature aging or susceptibility to age-related diseases, effectively shortening life. Conversely, other genes appear to promote resilience and longevity. Populations with a higher prevalence of such "longevity genes" often exhibit more centenarians, or individuals who live to be 100 or older.

Epigenetics: The Dynamic Layer

While our DNA sequence provides the primary script of life, it doesn't tell the whole story. This is where epigenetics comes in. Epigenetics refers to modifications on or around the DNA that affect gene activity without altering the DNA sequence itself.

Epigenetic changes, such as DNA methylation or histone modifications, act as regulators, determining which genes are turned on or off in a particular cell at a given time. Think of genetics as the keys of a piano and epigenetics as the pianist, deciding which keys to press or release to produce a melody.

The dynamic nature of epigenetics allows our genes to respond to the environment. Factors like diet, stress, physical activity, and even toxins can bring about epigenetic changes that influence our health and longevity. For instance, smoking can introduce specific epigenetic modifications that increase the risk of various diseases, potentially reducing lifespan.

The Interplay: Genetics, Epigenetics, and Aging

Genetics sets the stage, providing the potential for lifespan based on our inherited genes. Epigenetics, influenced by both genetics and the environment, modulates this potential throughout our lives. Together, they shape the trajectory of aging.

One compelling illustration of this interplay is the "epigenetic clock." Scientists have discovered specific patterns of DNA methylation that correlate with age. More fascinating is that this "biological age" determined by the epigenetic clock can differ from one's chronological age. Those with a "younger" biological age often enjoy better health and live longer, even if their chronological age is higher.

Influencing Longevity: Is It All Predestined?

While genes play an undeniable role in longevity, they aren't the sole determinants. Studies on identical twins, who share the same genetic makeup, have revealed that they can have different lifespans and health trajectories. This variance is often attributed to differences in their epigenomes, which can be influenced by individual experiences, choices, and environments.

The dynamic nature of epigenetics offers a glimmer of hope. It suggests that, to some extent, we can influence our health and potentially our longevity. Lifestyle choices that promote positive epigenetic changes, such as a balanced diet, regular exercise, and stress management, might pave the way for a longer, healthier life.

Future Prospects: Can We "Edit" Longevity?

With our expanding understanding of genetics and epigenetics, there's a tantalizing possibility on the horizon: the ability to intervene in the aging process. If specific genes or epigenetic patterns promote longevity, can we modify or leverage them?

Indeed, some strategies are already being explored. For instance, drugs that target epigenetic enzymes are being studied for their potential to rejuvenate cells or combat age-related diseases. Genetic therapies, too, might someday correct mutations that predispose individuals to premature aging or age-related conditions.

However, such interventions come with ethical, safety, and practical considerations. The prospect of "editing" longevity also raises profound questions about the nature of life, societal implications, and what it truly means to age gracefully.

In Conclusion

The intricate dance between genetics and epigenetics plays a foundational role in determining longevity. While genetics offers a glimpse into our potential lifespan, epigenetics modulates this potential in response to our environment and choices. Together, they weave the tapestry of our lives, influencing how we age and how long we live.

As we stand on the cusp of revolutionary biological insights, the domains of genetics and epigenetics offer not just understanding but also hope — the hope that we might one day harness this knowledge to extend health and life, ensuring that our later years are as golden as our youth.

Chapter 1: Basics of Epigenetics

Definition and History of Epigenetics

Epigenetics is a rapidly expanding field, providing fresh insights into our understanding of biology, inheritance, and gene regulation. However, to fully appreciate its significance, it's essential to trace its origins and understand its core definitions.

Defining Epigenetics

Epigenetics, at its heart, refers to the study of changes in organisms caused by modifications of gene expression rather than alterations of the genetic code itself. In other words, while the DNA sequence remains unchanged, the way genes are expressed— whether they're turned "on" or "off"—can be altered through epigenetic modifications.

The term "epigenetics" is derived from the Greek "epi-", meaning "above" or "on top of." So, epigenetics deals with molecular events "on top of" or "in addition to" the traditional genetic basis for inheritance.

Epigenetic modifications often involve chemical tags added to DNA or its associated proteins, dictating how genes are read by the cell. These changes can be transient or, in some cases, persist over multiple generations.

The Origins of Epigenetics

While epigenetics feels like a modern concept, its roots trace back to early 20th century developmental biology. The term "epigenesis" was initially used to describe the process by which a complex multicellular organism develops from a fertilized egg.

It was the British developmental biologist Conrad Waddington in the 1940s who coined the term "epigenetics." He used it to conceptualize how genes might interact with their surroundings to produce a phenotype—an organism's observable traits. Waddington famously visualized this process as a ball rolling down a contoured landscape, called an "epigenetic landscape." Each route the ball could take represented a different developmental pathway.

The Molecular Era

The true molecular understanding of epigenetics began to unfold in the latter half of the 20th century. As molecular biology techniques advanced, researchers began to observe that DNA in cells was not naked, but rather wrapped around proteins called histones. These histones could undergo chemical modifications, influencing gene expression.

By the 1970s and 1980s, scientists were discovering that the DNA itself could also be chemically modified, most notably by the addition of methyl groups—a process known as DNA methylation. These methylation patterns were seen to play critical roles in gene regulation, cellular differentiation, and even the inactivation of one X chromosome in female mammals.

The Contemporary Understanding

The turn of the 21st century witnessed an explosion of interest in epigenetics, fueled by technological advancements and the completion of the Human Genome Project. With the entire human DNA sequence mapped, attention shifted from "what is the sequence?" to "how is it regulated?"

This period saw the discovery of molecules like small RNA species that, while not coding for proteins, played pivotal roles in gene regulation. Such non-coding RNAs added another layer to the epigenetic regulation tapestry.

Additionally, the realization that epigenetic changes were reversible opened up therapeutic possibilities. If diseases were caused by epigenetic errors, could they be treated by "resetting" these changes?

Epigenetics Beyond Humans

While much of the focus in epigenetics has centered on human biology, it's crucial to recognize its broader applicability. Plants, for instance, heavily rely on epigenetic mechanisms, especially since they cannot "escape" their environment and must adapt in place. Studies on plants have provided critical insights into epigenetic processes like RNA-directed DNA methylation.

Similarly, in the realm of microbiology, epigenetic-like processes have been observed in bacteria, playing roles in processes like antibiotic resistance—a pressing concern in modern medicine.

Challenges and Evolving Definitions

It's worth noting that the definition of epigenetics has been a point of contention. As our understanding deepens and broadens, definitions evolve. While the core concept revolves around heritable changes not involving DNA sequence alterations, debates continue about what precisely falls under the epigenetic umbrella, especially when discussing transgenerational epigenetic inheritance.

In Conclusion

From its embryonic roots in developmental biology to its contemporary significance in therapeutics, epigenetics has traveled a remarkable journey. It serves as a testament to the layered complexity of life, reminding us that the code of life, the DNA, is just the beginning of the story. How this code is interpreted, edited, and expressed is where epigenetics shines, offering insights into the very fabric of life, development, and inheritance.

Key Concepts: DNA Methylation, Histone Modification, and Non-Coding RNA

The realm of epigenetics is vast and multi-faceted, but three principal mechanisms dominate the landscape: DNA methylation, histone modification, and the actions of non-coding RNAs. These are the molecular tools that cells use to regulate gene expression, ensuring that genes are active or silent when needed, contributing to the immense diversity of cell types and functions.

DNA Methylation: The Molecular "Off Switch"

Definition: DNA methylation is the addition of a methyl group (CH_3) to the cytosine base of DNA. This modification typically occurs at regions called CpG dinucleotides, where a cytosine is located next to a guanine base.

Role in gene regulation: DNA methylation is often associated with the repression of gene expression. When DNA is methylated at gene promoters (regions controlling gene expression), it often hinders the binding of transcriptional machinery, thereby silencing the gene. DNA methylation is crucial for processes like cellular differentiation, X-chromosome inactivation in females, and genomic imprinting, where genes are expressed based on their parent of origin.

Dynamics: DNA methylation patterns are established by enzymes called DNA methyltransferases. These patterns are not static but can change in response to environmental signals or during different developmental stages.

Histone Modification: The Dynamic Sculptors of Chromatin

Definition: Histones are proteins around which DNA is wound, forming a structure called chromatin. The DNA-histone interaction can be altered by adding or removing chemical groups to histones, such as methyl, acetyl, or phosphate groups. These changes are collectively termed histone modifications.

Role in gene regulation: Depending on the type and location of the histone modification, gene expression can be either upregulated or downregulated. For instance:

- **Histone acetylation:** Typically found at lysine residues on histones, acetylation often relaxes the chromatin structure, making the DNA more accessible to transcriptional machinery, promoting gene expression.

- **Histone methylation:** Can either activate or repress gene transcription depending on the specific lysine residue modified and the number of methyl groups added. For example, tri-methylation at lysine 27 on histone 3 (H3K27me3) is associated with gene repression, while tri-methylation at lysine 4 on histone 3 (H3K4me3) is linked to gene activation.

Dynamics: Enzymes responsible for adding (writers), removing (erasers), and reading (readers) histone modifications ensure dynamic regulation. This flexibility allows cells to swiftly respond to various stimuli, ensuring appropriate gene expression.

Non-Coding RNA: Silent Sequences with Loud Impacts

Definition: Not all RNA molecules serve as templates for protein synthesis. Non-coding RNAs (ncRNAs) are RNA molecules that don't code for proteins but have critical roles in regulating various cellular processes.

Role in gene regulation: There are numerous types of ncRNAs, each with unique functions:

- **microRNAs (miRNAs):** Small RNA molecules that can bind to messenger RNAs (mRNAs) and inhibit their translation or lead to their degradation. They act as post-transcriptional regulators of gene expression.

- **long non-coding RNAs (lncRNAs):** Larger RNA molecules with diverse roles, including serving as scaffolds that recruit chromatin-modifying enzymes, influencing histone modifications, or interacting with transcription factors to modulate their activity.

- **Piwi-interacting RNAs (piRNAs):** Associated with the Piwi class of proteins, they play essential roles in maintaining genome stability in germline cells.

Dynamics: The expression of ncRNAs can be tissue-specific, developmental stage-specific, or altered in diseases. Their dynamic expression patterns allow them to fine-tune gene regulation, ensuring cellular homeostasis.

Bringing It All Together

While DNA methylation, histone modification, and non-coding RNAs can operate independently, they often interplay, creating an intricate regulatory network. For instance, certain lncRNAs can recruit enzymes responsible for DNA methylation or histone modification, creating an epigenetic landscape conducive for gene silencing.

Understanding these key concepts is essential, as they underpin the myriad ways cells regulate gene expression, ensuring that genes are expressed in the right place, at the right time, and in the right amount.

The Dynamic Nature of the Epigenome

While the genome—a complete set of DNA in an organism—remains largely static throughout an individual's life, the epigenome is a living, breathing entity. Unlike the fixed sequence of nucleotide bases in DNA, the epigenome is ever-changing, responding to a host of internal and external cues. This dynamic nature plays a central role in development, adaptation, and even the potential for disease.

Epigenetic Plasticity: A Double-Edged Sword

The ability of the epigenome to change is both a blessing and a curse. On the one hand, it enables adaptability. Cells can react to environmental changes, developmental cues, or shifts in cellular function by adjusting gene expression without altering the underlying DNA. On the other hand, this plasticity can become problematic when dysregulated, leading to inappropriate gene expression patterns that can contribute to diseases like cancer.

Influences Shaping the Epigenome

1. Developmental Cues

From a single fertilized egg, a complex organism with myriad cell types arises, each with a distinct function. The journey involves cells "deciding" their fate, a process driven largely by the epigenome.

- **Cell differentiation:** As cells move down specific developmental pathways, the epigenome ensures that genes necessary for a cell's function are active, while others are silenced. For instance, a liver cell will have genes related to liver function activated but will silence genes associated with, say, neuron function.

- **Tissue-specific patterns:** Different tissues have characteristic epigenetic profiles, which are crucial for tissue identity and function.

2. Environmental Factors

The epigenome is sensitive to external conditions, acting as a bridge between the environment and the genetic blueprint.

- **Diet:** Nutrients can influence the availability of molecules needed for epigenetic modifications. For instance, a diet rich in folate and other methyl donors can affect DNA methylation patterns.

- **Toxins:** Exposure to certain toxins can modify the epigenome, potentially leading to diseases. For example, tobacco smoke has been shown to induce specific epigenetic changes associated with cancer risk.

- **Stress:** Psychological and physical stressors can leave epigenetic marks, impacting health outcomes. Prenatal stress, in particular, can have long-lasting epigenetic effects on the developing fetus.

3. Aging

As organisms age, the epigenome undergoes shifts, some of which are associated with age-related diseases and declining cellular function. These changes can include altered DNA methylation patterns and changes in histone modifications.

Memory of the Epigenome: Transgenerational Epigenetic Inheritance

One of the most intriguing aspects of the dynamic epigenome is its potential to pass on information to subsequent generations. While the traditional Mendelian principles of inheritance focus on the transmission of DNA sequences, there's accumulating evidence suggesting that epigenetic changes in one generation can affect the next.

- **Famine studies:** Historical events like the Dutch Hunger Winter during World War II provided evidence that malnutrition in pregnant mothers led to health effects not just in their children but also in subsequent generations, hinting at the role of epigenetics.
- **Model organisms:** Experiments in organisms like plants, worms, and mice have shown that certain epigenetic changes can persist for several generations.

However, the mechanisms and extent of transgenerational epigenetic inheritance in humans remain a topic of intense research and debate.

Epigenetic Resets

While the epigenome is dynamic, it also undergoes global "resets" during specific developmental stages:

- **Primordial germ cells:** These cells, which give rise to sperm and eggs, undergo extensive epigenetic reprogramming, erasing most of the epigenetic marks to ensure a clean slate for the next generation.
- **Early embryogenesis:** After fertilization, the developing embryo undergoes significant epigenetic changes, setting the stage for subsequent developmental processes.

These resets underscore the importance of epigenetic regulation during development and the potential implications of any disruptions in this intricate process.

Concluding Thoughts

The dynamic nature of the epigenome is a testament to the complex interplay between genes and the environment. It adds layers of regulatory control, ensuring that organisms can adapt, develop, and function optimally. However, with this dynamism comes vulnerability. Disruptions in the delicate balance of the epigenome can pave the way for disease, emphasizing the importance of understanding and potentially harnessing epigenetic processes for therapeutic interventions.

Chapter 2:
The Epigenetic Clock

Introduction to the Concept of Biological vs. Chronological Age

Aging, a universal phenomenon, touches every living organism. However, how we perceive age and how it manifests biologically are multifaceted concepts. At the core of understanding age lies the distinction between "chronological" and "biological" age. This distinction offers a deeper insight into health, longevity, and the intricate dance between our genes and the environment.

Chronological Age: The Inevitable Passage of Time

Definition: Chronological age represents the actual time an individual has been alive—it's as simple as counting the number of years since one's birth.

- **Uniform progression:** Regardless of lifestyle, genetics, or environmental exposures, one's chronological age progresses uniformly—one year per year.

- **Legal and social implications:** Chronological age has significant societal implications. It dictates when one can vote, retire, or be considered an adult or senior. Societal norms and laws are often structured around this tangible measure of age.

Biological Age: A Reflection of Internal Wear and Tear

Definition: In contrast, biological age reflects an individual's physiological and cellular state. It captures how well or how poorly the body's systems are functioning compared to a typical benchmark, often corresponding to chronological age.

- **Variable progression:** Unlike the steadfast march of chronological age, biological age can vary widely among individuals
  of the same chronological age. Some might show advanced
  signs of cellular aging and related health issues, while others
  remain youthful and vibrant.

- **Influencing factors:** A myriad of elements can influence
  biological age, including genetics, lifestyle choices (like diet,
  exercise, and smoking), exposure to environmental toxins,
  and more.

Why the Distinction Matters

Understanding the difference between these two concepts of age
is paramount for several reasons:

1. **Health assessment:** While chronological age can suggest susceptibility to certain age-related diseases, biological age provides a more precise measure. Two individuals, both 60 years
   old chronologically, might have different risks for diseases like
   heart disease or dementia based on their biological ages.

2. **Aging interventions:** If we can assess biological age, we can
   potentially intervene to slow its progression. This notion
   forms the foundation of numerous anti-aging research efforts
   and therapies.

3. **Personalized medicine:** Recognizing the differences between
   chronological and biological age can lead to more personalized healthcare strategies. Interventions, preventative measures, or treatments could be tailored based on an individual's biological age rather than their chronological age.

The Epigenetic Connection

One of the most promising markers for biological age lies in the
realm of epigenetics. The patterns of chemical modifications on
DNA, particularly DNA methylation, have been found to change
with age. These changes are so consistent that researchers have
developed "epigenetic clocks" that can predict an individual's age
with remarkable accuracy. But more importantly, these clocks can

provide insights into an individual's biological age and their risk for various age-related ailments.

Horvath's Clock: One of the most well-known epigenetic clocks was developed by Dr. Steve Horvath. By assessing methylation patterns at specific DNA sites, this clock can predict chronological age. Deviations from the predicted age can suggest accelerated or decelerated biological aging.

The beauty of epigenetic clocks lies in their potential to be more than just predictors of age. They could provide insights into why some individuals age faster or slower than others and offer avenues for interventions that promote healthy aging.

Concluding Thoughts

Age, as a concept, is more profound than the mere passage of time. While we all move uniformly in chronological age, our bodies narrate different tales of time's impact. The divergence between chronological and biological age offers a window into the complexity of aging, the factors that drive it, and the potential to influence its trajectory. As we delve deeper into the intricacies of the epigenetic clock in subsequent sections, we'll uncover the molecular intricacies of aging and the promise they hold for a future of healthy longevity.

The Science Behind DNA Methylation as a Predictor of Age

The quest to understand and quantify aging has led researchers down various avenues of biological investigation. Among these, DNA methylation stands out as a particularly compelling marker, offering a window into the molecular processes of aging and the potential to predict chronological and biological age with remarkable precision.

DNA Methylation: A Brief Overview

Before delving into its relationship with aging, it's crucial to understand what DNA methylation is.

- **Definition:** DNA methylation is a chemical modification where a methyl group (-CH3) is added to the cytosine base of DNA, typically at a CpG dinucleotide site (where a cytosine nucleotide is immediately followed by a guanine nucleotide).

- **Role:** Methylation plays a critical role in regulating gene expression. When a gene promoter region is methylated, it often leads to the repression of gene transcription, effectively "silencing" the gene.

Methylation Patterns and Aging

The methylation status of many CpG sites in the genome changes predictably with age. As individuals grow older, some regions of the genome become increasingly methylated, while others become less so.

- **Global vs. site-specific changes:** While there's a general decrease in global DNA methylation with age, specific CpG sites show increased methylation. These site-specific changes are of particular interest in developing epigenetic clocks.

- **Consistency across individuals:** The predictability of age-related methylation changes is surprisingly consistent across individuals, making it a robust marker for age estimation.

Development of the Epigenetic Clock

Using the age-associated patterns of DNA methylation, researchers have developed algorithms to predict an individual's age. These algorithms, or "epigenetic clocks," use the methylation status of specific CpG sites to estimate age.

- **Horvath's Clock:** Dr. Steve Horvath's epigenetic clock, one of the most widely recognized, uses methylation data from 353 CpG sites. This clock can predict chronological age across various tissues and cell types, with an astonishing accuracy of 2.9 years on average.

- **Hannum's Clock:** Developed around the same time as Horvath's, this clock is based on methylation patterns in 71 CpG sites and was initially developed using whole blood samples.

Beyond Chronological Age: Indications of Biological Aging

While predicting chronological age is impressive in itself, the true potential of DNA methylation patterns lies in their ability to reflect biological age.

- **Age acceleration:** If the predicted age from an epigenetic clock is higher than the chronological age, it indicates accelerated aging. Conversely, a predicted age lower than the chronological age suggests decelerated aging.

- **Associations with health outcomes:** Age acceleration, as indicated by methylation patterns, has been associated with various age-related diseases, cognitive decline, and even mortality. For instance, individuals with accelerated aging based on methylation patterns have a higher risk of developing conditions like Alzheimer's disease.

Mechanisms: Why Does DNA Methylation Change with Age?

While the association between DNA methylation and age is evident, the underlying mechanisms driving these changes remain a subject of ongoing research.

- **Cumulative effects of the environment:** One theory suggests that over time, environmental factors, such as exposure to toxins, diet, and lifestyle choices, lead to the accumulation of methylation changes.

- **Cellular processes:** Intrinsic cellular processes, like DNA replication errors or the production of reactive oxygen species, may contribute to changes in DNA methylation over time.

- **Stem cell differentiation:** As stem cells differentiate and renew over an individual's lifespan, shifts in their methylation patterns might contribute to the overall age-related changes observed.

Concluding Thoughts

The exploration of DNA methylation as an age predictor underscores the molecular intricacies of the aging process. The epigenetic clock, rooted in methylation patterns, offers more than just a glimpse into one's chronological age—it provides insights into health, potential disease risk, and the broader mysteries of longevity. As research in this realm advances, there's hope that understanding and perhaps even manipulating these epigenetic changes could pave the way for interventions that promote healthy aging and extend lifespan.

Implications for Health and Lifespan Predictions

The intricate dance of DNA methylation patterns with age does more than serve as a chronometer for our cells. The epigenetic clock, as read through methylation markers, holds profound implications for our health, disease susceptibility, and even potential lifespan. As we delve into the deeper ramifications of this molecular timekeeper, we uncover an array of possibilities for personalized medicine, early interventions, and improved health outcomes.

Health Indicators and the Epigenetic Clock

The degree to which one's predicted epigenetic age deviates from their chronological age—often termed "epigenetic age acceleration"—can serve as an important health indicator.

- **Disease susceptibility:** Numerous studies have linked epigenetic age acceleration to a higher risk for various age-associated diseases, from cardiovascular disorders to neurodegenerative conditions like Alzheimer's. People with a higher epigenetic age relative to their chronological age might be at a heightened risk for these diseases.

- **Cognitive and physical health:** Accelerated epigenetic aging has also been associated with cognitive decline and poorer physical health. This link underscores the importance of the epigenetic clock in holistic health assessment, spanning both mental and physical domains.

Predicting Lifespan: Beyond Just Age

While age prediction is valuable, another tantalizing potential of the epigenetic clock lies in its ability to predict lifespan.

- **Mortality risk:** Some studies suggest that individuals with a higher epigenetic age (relative to chronological age) might face an increased risk of mortality. This means that the epigenetic clock could potentially provide insights into an individual's expected healthspan and lifespan.
- **Biomarker for interventions:** By monitoring how certain interventions—ranging from dietary changes to drug therapies—affect the epigenetic clock, researchers might be able to gauge the potential of these interventions to extend lifespan or improve healthspan.

Personalized Medicine and the Promise of Early Interventions

With the knowledge gained from the epigenetic clock, there emerges an opportunity to craft more personalized and timely health interventions.

- **Tailored health strategies:** If an individual is identified as having an accelerated epigenetic age, healthcare providers might recommend specific strategies or treatments tailored to mitigate the associated risks.
- **Early interventions:** One of the most powerful applications of the epigenetic clock is the potential for early intervention. Before the onset of symptomatic diseases, adjustments in lifestyle, diet, or therapeutic interventions might be initiated to decelerate the aging process and ward off potential diseases.

Potential Modifiers of the Epigenetic Clock

Understanding the factors that influence the progression of the epigenetic clock can provide pathways for interventions.

- **Lifestyle factors:** Smoking, alcohol consumption, physical activity, and dietary habits have all been explored for their influence on the epigenetic clock. For instance, prolonged smoking has been associated with accelerated epigenetic aging.

- **Environmental exposures:** Chronic exposures to certain environmental factors, such as toxins or pollutants, might accelerate the epigenetic clock. Conversely, positive environmental factors, such as engagement in mentally stimulating activities, could potentially decelerate the clock.

- **Genetics:** While the epigenome reflects the influence of environmental factors on gene function, genetics still play a role. Some individuals might be genetically predisposed to have an epigenome that's more resilient to age-accelerating factors.

Ethical Considerations: The Double-Edged Sword

As with any powerful tool, the insights gained from the epigenetic clock come with ethical considerations.

- **Privacy concerns:** As epigenetic data can reveal intimate details about an individual's health and potential lifespan, ensuring the privacy and security of this information is paramount.

- **Potential for discrimination:** There's a risk that epigenetic age data could be used discriminatorily, especially by insurance companies in assessing coverage or premiums.

- **Emotional impact:** Knowing one's epigenetic age and its associated risks can have significant emotional implications. Proper counseling and support should accompany any discussions related to these insights.

Concluding Thoughts

The intertwining of our epigenome with the tapestry of age paints a vivid picture of health, potential, and the myriad factors that influence our journey through time. As we harness the insights of the epigenetic clock, we're bestowed with the power—and responsibility—to shape healthier, longer lives, armed with knowledge and precision.

Chapter 3: Lifestyle and the Epigenome

Diet and its Impact on DNA Methylation Patterns

Diet, one of the most fundamental aspects of our daily lives, extends its influence far beyond mere sustenance. Every food choice we make holds the potential to impact our cells, particularly our epigenome. Among the myriad of epigenetic modifications, DNA methylation stands out as particularly sensitive to dietary influences. This section delves into the profound relationship between our dietary habits and the methylation patterns etched onto our DNA.

The Dynamic Interplay: Nutrients and DNA Methylation

The food we consume is a rich source of molecules that can either directly or indirectly influence DNA methylation.

- **Methyl donors:** Foods rich in methyl groups play a direct role in DNA methylation. Essential nutrients like folate, choline, and methionine are primary methyl donors. They contribute to the production of S-adenosylmethionine (SAM), a principal molecule responsible for transferring methyl groups during the methylation process.

- **Bioactive compounds:** Beyond just methyl donors, various bioactive compounds found in food can influence DNA methylation either by modulating enzymes that add or remove methyl groups or by affecting the availability of SAM.

Specific Foods and their Epigenetic Impact

Numerous dietary components have been studied for their effects on DNA methylation, with some of the most noteworthy being:

- **Green tea:** Epigallocatechin-3-gallate (EGCG), a major component of green tea, has been found to influence DNA methylation by inhibiting the DNA methyltransferase enzyme. This can potentially reactivate genes that have been silenced by methylation.

- **Soy products:** Soy is rich in isoflavones like genistein, which can modulate DNA methylation. This modulation might partly explain the potential protective effects of soy against certain cancers.

- **Cruciferous vegetables:** Compounds like sulforaphane, found in broccoli and other cruciferous vegetables, have been shown to influence DNA methylation patterns, potentially playing a role in cancer prevention.

- **Alcohol:** Chronic alcohol consumption can lead to aberrant DNA methylation patterns, potentially contributing to the development of diseases like cancer.

Diet-Induced Methylation Changes: Health Implications

Changes in DNA methylation patterns induced by diet can have profound health consequences, especially when they alter gene expression in critical pathways.

- **Cancer:** Diet-induced changes in DNA methylation can influence the expression of tumor suppressor genes or oncogenes, potentially playing a role in cancer initiation, progression, or resistance to therapy.

- **Cardiovascular disease:** Nutrient imbalance can lead to changes in DNA methylation patterns associated with inflammation, cholesterol metabolism, and vascular health.

- **Neurodegenerative diseases:** Diet can impact the methylation of genes involved in neurological functions, potentially influencing the risk of conditions like Alzheimer's disease.

The Lifelong Influence of Early Diet

The influence of diet on DNA methylation isn't limited to adult-hood. Early-life nutrition, starting from the prenatal period, can leave lasting marks on the epigenome.

- **Fetal programming:** Nutrient availability during critical periods of fetal development can influence DNA methylation patterns in ways that predispose individuals to diseases later in life, a phenomenon termed "fetal programming."
- **Breastfeeding and infant nutrition:** Breast milk is a rich source of bioactive compounds that can influence the infant's epigenome. Moreover, early introduction or lack of certain foods can lead to epigenetic modifications with potential long-term health implications.

Personalized Nutrition: Tailoring Diet for the Epigenome

Understanding the epigenetic consequences of diet opens the door for personalized nutrition strategies.

- **Epigenetic testing:** By analyzing an individual's epigenetic markers, it might be possible to recommend specific dietary interventions tailored to their unique methylation patterns.
- **Dietary interventions:** For individuals with known health risks, targeted dietary changes can be used as interventions to potentially modify DNA methylation patterns in a beneficial manner.

Concluding Thoughts

The intricate dance between diet and DNA methylation showcases the profound ways in which our daily choices shape our health at the molecular level. As we continue to unravel the complexities of this relationship, we inch closer to harnessing the power of diet not just for nourishment, but for targeted epigenetic modulation, disease prevention, and health optimization.

Exercise and Epigenetic Age Reversal

The myriad benefits of exercise are well-known, from improved cardiovascular health to enhanced cognitive function. However, the influence of physical activity extends beyond the visible, leaving its mark at the cellular and molecular levels. Specifically, exercise holds a promising key to modulating the epigenome and potentially reversing epigenetic age. Let's dive into the transformative relationship between physical activity and epigenetic modifications.

Physical Activity: A Catalyst for Epigenetic Change

At the heart of exercise's influence on the epigenome is its ability to induce physiological stress, thereby triggering a cascade of cellular responses.

- **Stress and adaptation:** Exercise imposes stress on various bodily systems, prompting them to adapt. This adaptation, in turn, requires gene expression changes which are often mediated by epigenetic modifications, including DNA methylation, histone modifications, and non-coding RNAs.

- **Tissue-specific modifications:** Different types of exercise can lead to tissue-specific epigenetic changes. For instance, resistance training might primarily influence muscle tissue, while aerobic exercise may have pronounced effects on the cardiovascular system.

The Epigenetic Clock and Exercise: Turning Back Time?

Emerging research suggests that consistent physical activity can influence the epigenetic clock, possibly decelerating or even reversing epigenetic aging.

- **DNA methylation patterns:** Regular exercise has been shown to modify DNA methylation patterns in genes associated with aging and age-related diseases. This can potentially slow the progression of the epigenetic clock or bring it more in line with chronological age.

- **Histone modifications:** Exercise also impacts the configuration of histones, proteins around which DNA is wound. Specific modifications can activate or suppress genes related to longevity and healthspan.

How Exercise Might Reset the Clock

Several mechanisms through which exercise might influence the epigenetic clock have been proposed:

- **Anti-inflammatory effects:** Chronic inflammation is associated with accelerated epigenetic aging. Exercise reduces systemic inflammation, potentially influencing DNA methylation patterns associated with aging.

- **Enhanced autophagy:** Exercise promotes cellular cleanup processes like autophagy, where cells remove damaged components. Enhanced autophagy could potentially influence the epigenetic landscape and slow aging.

- **Improved mitochondrial function:** Physical activity boosts mitochondrial health and biogenesis. Since mitochondria play a pivotal role in cellular aging, their enhanced function might influence the epigenetic clock.

- **Hormonal modulation:** Exercise affects various hormones, including those linked with longevity, such as insulin-like growth factor (IGF-1) and growth hormone. Hormonal changes can, in turn, mediate epigenetic modifications.

Exercise Intensity, Duration, and Type: Finding the Sweet Spot

Not all exercise is created equal when it comes to epigenetic influence.

- **Aerobic vs. anaerobic:** While both types of exercise impart beneficial epigenetic changes, they might target different sets of genes. Aerobic activities, such as running or swimming, often have more pronounced effects on cardiovascular health, while anaerobic activities, like weightlifting, may impact muscle-associated genes more prominently.

- **Duration and frequency:** The cumulative effects of exercise over time seem to be crucial for epigenetic benefits. Short bursts of intense activity might trigger immediate epigenetic changes, but sustained activity over months or years appears to have a more lasting impact on the epigenetic clock.
- **Age and exercise:** The age at which one begins consistent exercise might influence its epigenetic impact. Early-life physical activity could set a foundation for a healthier epigenome, but even initiating exercise in later life holds benefits.

Health Implications: Beyond Just Feeling Younger

The potential age-reversing effects of exercise at the epigenetic level have profound health implications:

- **Disease prevention:** By influencing genes associated with age-related diseases, exercise could reduce the risk of conditions like heart disease, diabetes, and neurodegenerative diseases.
- **Cognitive health:** Physical activity has been shown to influence the epigenetic patterns of genes involved in brain function, possibly delaying cognitive decline and reducing the risk of conditions like Alzheimer's.
- **Improved longevity:** While more research is needed, the potential for exercise to slow or reverse epigenetic aging suggests that it might play a role in extending not just healthspan but lifespan as well.

Concluding Thoughts

The adage "move it or lose it" gains profound depth when viewed through the lens of epigenetics. Exercise, in its myriad forms, emerges as a potent tool in our arsenal against the inexorable march of time, offering the tantalizing possibility of not just slowing the clock but, at the molecular level, turning it back.

The Epigenetic Consequences of Smoking, Alcohol, and Stress

The lifestyle choices we make, often driven by societal norms or personal circumstances, can leave indelible marks on our epigenome. Three prominent lifestyle factors – smoking, alcohol consumption, and chronic stress – exert profound epigenetic effects that can influence our health and longevity. Delving into these relationships provides crucial insights into the silent cellular repercussions of our daily habits.

Smoking: A Cloud of Epigenetic Alterations

Long-established as a leading cause of preventable diseases, tobacco smoking is not just harmful at the physiological level. It instigates a cascade of epigenetic changes that can persist even after smoking cessation.

- **DNA methylation:** Smoking has been linked to altered DNA methylation patterns across numerous genes. Some genes become hypermethylated (gaining methylation marks) leading to their silencing, while others become hypomethylated (losing methylation marks) leading to their activation.

- **Histone modifications:** Exposure to cigarette smoke can influence the configuration of histones, altering gene expression patterns in ways that can promote disease.

- **Implications for health:** The epigenetic changes induced by smoking have been linked to various diseases, including cancers (especially lung cancer), cardiovascular diseases, and respiratory conditions.

- **Reversibility:** Interestingly, while some epigenetic marks induced by smoking appear to be reversible upon cessation, others might persist for years, emphasizing the lasting impact of smoking on the epigenome.

Alcohol: Beyond the Buzz to the Epigenome

Moderate alcohol consumption is often perceived as benign or even beneficial. However, chronic excessive drinking can have dire epigenetic consequences.

- **DNA methylation patterns:** Chronic alcohol intake has been linked to widespread changes in DNA methylation, especially in genes associated with liver function, increasing the risk of liver diseases.
- **Histone modifications:** Alcohol can alter the acetylation and methylation status of histones, affecting genes involved in addiction pathways and increasing the risk of developing alcohol use disorders.
- **Non-coding RNAs:** Alcohol influences the expression of various non-coding RNAs, which can modulate the expression of genes involved in inflammation, liver function, and neuronal health.
- **Implications for health:** Beyond liver diseases, the epigenetic changes induced by alcohol can increase the risk of cancers, heart diseases, and neurodegenerative conditions.

Stress: Silent Cellular Strains

While acute stress can be adaptive, chronic stress, whether psychological or physiological, can wreak havoc on our epigenome.

- **Glucocorticoid receptor genes:** Chronic stress leads to altered methylation patterns in the genes for glucocorticoid receptors, affecting how individuals respond to future stressors.
- **Brain-derived neurotrophic factor (BDNF):** Stress can influence the methylation of the BDNF gene, which plays a crucial role in neuronal health and plasticity. Altered BDNF expression has implications for mood disorders and cognitive function.
- **Telomeres and stress:** Chronic stress has been linked to shortened telomeres, the protective caps on chromosomes. While not a direct epigenetic modification, telomere length is influenced by epigenetic factors and is an indicator of cellular aging.

- **Implications for health:** The epigenetic modifications induced by chronic stress are linked to a plethora of health issues, including mental health disorders, cardiovascular diseases, metabolic disorders, and a weakened immune system.

Interplay and Cumulative Effects

While we've discussed these factors separately, it's crucial to understand that many individuals are simultaneously exposed to multiple lifestyle factors, leading to intertwined and cumulative epigenetic effects.

- **Combined effects:** The combined epigenetic impact of, say, smoking and alcohol can be more pronounced than either factor alone, potentially leading to an enhanced risk of diseases like cancers.

- **Individual variability:** Not everyone responds identically to these lifestyle factors. Genetic predispositions, early-life exposures, and other individual factors can modulate the epigenetic consequences of smoking, alcohol, and stress.

Concluding Thoughts

Our lifestyle choices, both conscious and imposed upon us, echo silently but persistently at the cellular level. Recognizing the epigenetic repercussions of habits like smoking, drinking, and enduring chronic stress underscores the need for proactive health strategies. As we deepen our understanding of these intricate epigenetic landscapes, we are better equipped to develop interventions that can mitigate or even reverse the detrimental marks left by these lifestyle factors.

Other Environmental Factors Influencing the Epigenome

While lifestyle choices like diet, exercise, smoking, and alcohol consumption have pronounced effects on the epigenome, various other environmental factors also play critical roles in shaping our epigenetic landscape. These factors, ranging from pollutants to early-life events, offer profound insights into the intricate dance between our environment and our genes.

Air Pollution: Beyond Breathing Difficulties

Air pollution, with its mixture of particulate matter, gases, and chemicals, doesn't just impact respiratory health but has far-reaching epigenetic implications.

- **DNA methylation changes:** Exposure to pollutants like polycyclic aromatic hydrocarbons (PAHs) has been linked to alterations in DNA methylation patterns, especially in genes associated with inflammation and immune responses.
- **Histone modifications:** Particulate matter and other pollutants can influence histone acetylation and methylation, affecting genes related to oxidative stress and cardiovascular function.
- **Health repercussions:** The epigenetic modifications due to air pollution increase the risk of respiratory diseases, cardiovascular conditions, and even neurodegenerative disorders.

Early-Life Exposures: Imprints that Last

Events and exposures during prenatal and early postnatal life can leave lasting epigenetic marks, influencing health outcomes decades later.

- **Fetal exposures:** Nutritional deficiencies, toxins, or stress experienced by a pregnant mother can alter the fetus's epigenetic patterns, predisposing the child to metabolic disorders, cardiovascular diseases, and even mental health issues.
- **Neonatal experiences:** Early life adversities, like malnutrition or trauma, can set epigenetic patterns that impact cognitive function, stress responses, and disease susceptibility later in life.

Pesticides, Plastics, and Chemicals: The Invisible Threats

Various chemicals that we encounter daily, often unbeknownst to us, can stealthily modify our epigenome.

- **Bisphenol A (BPA):** A common component in plastics, BPA exposure can lead to DNA methylation changes, particularly in genes related to hormonal pathways and reproduction.
- **Pesticides:** Many pesticides influence the epigenome, especially impacting genes related to neurological function and development.
- **Heavy metals:** Exposure to metals like arsenic, lead, and cadmium has been linked to widespread epigenetic changes, increasing the risk of cancers, cardiovascular diseases, and cognitive impairments.

Infections and the Immune Response

Pathogenic infections, whether viral, bacterial, or parasitic, can instigate a cascade of epigenetic modifications.

- **Viral infections:** Viruses like HIV, HPV, and the Epstein-Barr virus can modify host DNA methylation patterns and histone configurations to facilitate their replication or evade the immune response.
- **Bacterial infections:** Some bacteria release toxins that influence host epigenetic patterns or directly modify host DNA methylation to enhance their survival.
- **Implications for health:** These infection-induced epigenetic changes can predispose individuals to cancers, chronic inflammatory conditions, and other diseases.

Light and Circadian Rhythms: The Biological Clock's Influence

Our internal biological clocks, influenced by light exposure patterns, also modulate the epigenetic landscape.

- **Light exposure:** Chronic exposure to artificial light, especially at night, can alter DNA methylation patterns and histone configurations in genes related to the circadian rhythm.
- **Shift work:** Individuals engaged in shift work, with disrupted sleep patterns, often exhibit epigenetic changes that increase the risk of metabolic disorders, cardiovascular diseases, and cancers.

Epigenetic Memory and Transgenerational Effects

Interestingly, some epigenetic modifications, especially those induced by profound environmental stresses, can be transmitted to subsequent generations.

- **Famine and epigenetic memory:** Historical events like the Dutch Hunger Winter during WWII have shown that individuals exposed to famine in utero had specific DNA methylation changes, some of which were also observed in their offspring.
- **Toxin exposure:** Certain toxins, when encountered by one generation, can induce epigenetic changes that persist in their descendants, predisposing them to various health issues.

Concluding Thoughts

Our environment, in its vast expanse of factors, constantly converses with our genes. This dialogue, often silent and imperceptible, shapes our epigenetic landscape, influencing not just our health but potentially the health of future generations. As we unravel these intricate epigenetic webs woven by environmental factors, we are better positioned to navigate our environment judiciously, advocating for cleaner, healthier spaces that foster well-being at the very core of our cellular existence.

Chapter 4: Caloric Restriction and Epigenetic Longevity

Overview of Caloric Restriction Studies Across Species

Caloric restriction (CR), the reduction of calorie intake without malnutrition, has been a focal point of longevity research for several decades. The consistent finding, transcending species boundaries, is that a reduction in caloric intake can significantly extend lifespan. But how does CR impart these benefits, and what can studies across various organisms tell us about its potential applicability to humans? Let's dive into an overview of CR's impact on diverse species and its intertwined relationship with the epigenome.

Yeast: Simplicity Lends Clarity

As one of the simplest organisms studied in the context of CR, yeast has provided foundational insights into the molecular mechanisms underpinning the longevity benefits of reduced calorie intake.

- **Lifespan extension:** CR, often achieved through glucose restriction, reliably extends the replicative lifespan of yeast.
- **Epigenetic underpinnings:** Histone deacetylases, such as Sir2, play a pivotal role in the lifespan-extending effects of CR in yeast, highlighting early connections between caloric intake, epigenetics, and longevity.

Worms and Flies: Small Organisms, Big Insights

C. elegans (a nematode) and Drosophila (fruit fly) have been stalwarts in aging research, with CR studies yielding enlightening findings.

- **Lifespan extension:** Both organisms exhibit extended lifespans under CR conditions, with C. elegans showing particularly robust responses to different dietary interventions.
- **Epigenetic alterations:** CR induces myriad epigenetic changes in these organisms, influencing histone modifications, DNA methylation patterns, and non-coding RNA expressions. These epigenetic shifts orchestrate protective cellular responses that enhance organismal longevity.

Mammalian Models: Rodents Lead the Way

Rodents, especially mice and rats, have been indispensable in translating CR findings to more complex organisms, providing clues about potential human implications.

- **Lifespan extension:** CR reliably extends the lifespan of various rodent species, reducing age-related pathologies like cancers, neurodegenerative diseases, and cardiovascular conditions.
- **Epigenetic dynamics:** The rodent epigenome is highly responsive to CR, with changes in DNA methylation, histone configurations, and non-coding RNA profiles. These epigenetic shifts influence genes associated with metabolism, inflammation, stress responses, and DNA repair, fostering a cellular environment conducive to longevity.

Non-human Primates: Closer to Home

Rhesus monkeys, due to their closer genetic kinship to humans, offer invaluable insights into CR's potential effects on human health and longevity.

- **Lifespan extension:** Long-term studies have shown that CR can extend the lifespan of rhesus monkeys while significantly reducing age-associated pathologies.

- **Epigenetic reflections:** While epigenetic studies in primates are still burgeoning, preliminary data suggest that CR modulates DNA methylation patterns and histone modifications in ways that mirror rodent findings. These epigenetic alterations are associated with enhanced metabolic health, reduced inflammation, and improved stress resistance.

Humans: Gleaning Insights from Limited Data

Direct, long-term CR studies in humans are logistically challenging and ethically complex. However, short-term studies and observations from specific populations provide some insights.

- **Health benefits:** Short-term CR studies in humans reveal improvements in cardiovascular health, metabolic markers, and reductions in markers of inflammation and oxidative stress.

- **Epigenetic indications:** While comprehensive epigenetic analyses post-CR in humans are scant, preliminary studies hint at changes in DNA methylation patterns, especially in genes associated with aging and age-related diseases.

Evolutionary Conservation: A Common Thread

One striking takeaway from CR studies across species is the evolutionary conservation of its benefits. From simple unicellular organisms to primates, the longevity and health-promoting effects of reduced caloric intake seem to be a fundamental biological principle.

- **Shared molecular pathways:** Several molecular pathways, such as those involving insulin/IGF-1 signaling, mTOR, and sirtuins, are influenced by CR across diverse species, hinting at common longevity mechanisms.

- **Epigenetic convergence:** The epigenetic changes induced by CR also exhibit remarkable similarities across species, underscoring the idea that epigenetic adaptations to reduced nutrient availability are evolutionarily conserved strategies to enhance survival.

Concluding Thoughts

Caloric restriction's ability to extend lifespan and promote health is a testament to the adaptive powers of organisms when faced with nutritional scarcity. As we unravel the epigenetic intricacies of this response, we inch closer to harnessing CR's benefits, potentially through interventions that mimic its effects without necessitating drastic dietary changes. The journey from yeast to humans paints a compelling narrative of resilience, adaptation, and the profound interplay between nutrition, epigenetics, and longevity.

Molecular Mechanisms Linking Restriction with Lifespan Extension

Caloric restriction (CR) is a powerful intervention that extends lifespan across a range of organisms, but how? Unraveling this question has led to fascinating discoveries about the molecular and cellular pathways influenced by reduced calorie intake. From signaling cascades to energy sensors and stress response pathways, let's delve into the intricate mechanisms through which CR influences health and longevity.

Insulin/IGF-1 Signaling: A Central Longevity Pathway

Insulin-like growth factor-1 (IGF-1) and insulin are vital players in nutrient sensing and growth regulation. It's no surprise that their pathways play a pivotal role in the longevity effects of CR.

- **Reduced signaling:** CR consistently reduces IGF-1 levels and insulin signaling, leading to a shift from growth and reproduction to maintenance and survival.

- **Lifespan extension:** In organisms like C. elegans, reduced insulin/IGF-1 signaling has been directly linked to longevity, with mutations in this pathway extending life.

- **Epigenetic crosstalk:** The insulin/IGF-1 pathway intersects with various epigenetic regulators, influencing gene expression patterns that bolster cellular resilience.

mTOR: Sensing Nutrients and Orchestrating Growth

The mechanistic target of rapamycin (mTOR) pathway is a central regulator of cellular growth, sensing amino acid and energy levels.

- **CR dampens mTOR signaling:** Under CR, reduced nutrient availability leads to suppressed mTOR activity, promoting longevity.

- **Health benefits:** Inhibition of mTOR, either through CR or drugs like rapamycin, extends lifespan in multiple organisms, while also protecting against age-related pathologies.

- **Epigenetic involvement:** mTOR interacts with various epigenetic processes, including histone modifications and the expression of non-coding RNAs, influencing genes related to growth, metabolism, and stress resistance.

Sirtuins: The Epigenetic Guardians of Longevity

Sirtuins, a family of NAD+-dependent protein deacetylases, emerge as essential mediators of CR's benefits, intertwining nutrient sensing with epigenetic regulation.

- **Activation by CR:** Reduced caloric intake boosts NAD+ levels, activating sirtuins, particularly SIRT1 in mammals.

- **Protective roles:** Activated sirtuins deacetylate numerous target proteins, bolstering DNA repair, suppressing inflammation, enhancing mitochondrial function, and promoting metabolic flexibility.

- **Direct epigenetic regulation:** Sirtuins directly influence chromatin structure by deacetylating histones, thereby modulating the transcriptional activity of genes crucial for longevity.

AMPK: The Cellular Energy Sensor

AMP-activated protein kinase (AMPK) serves as a central energy sensor, activated when cellular energy levels (ATP) are low, as seen during CR.

- **Activation by CR:** Reduced calorie intake elevates the AMP-to-ATP ratio, activating AMPK.
- **Promotion of catabolic processes:** Activated AMPK promotes energy-producing pathways, such as fatty acid oxidation and autophagy, while inhibiting energy-consuming processes like protein synthesis.
- **Epigenetic interplay:** AMPK influences various epigenetic enzymes, modulating DNA methylation, histone modifications, and the expression of non-coding RNAs, all of which can influence longevity-associated genes.

Enhanced Autophagy: Cellular Recycling at Its Best

Autophagy, a process where cells degrade and recycle damaged components, is another key mechanism through which CR promotes longevity.

- **Stimulation by CR:** Nutrient scarcity during CR triggers autophagy, allowing cells to maintain essential functions by recycling cellular materials.
- **Lifespan extension:** Enhanced autophagy is associated with increased lifespan and reduced age-related pathologies, as seen in multiple species.
- **Epigenetic regulation:** The autophagy machinery is, in part, regulated at the epigenetic level, with various histone modifications and non-coding RNAs modulating the expression of autophagy-related genes.

Enhanced Stress Resistance: Preparing for the Tough Times

CR induces a mild stress response, enhancing cellular resistance to more significant stresses, an effect known as hormesis.

- **Upregulation of stress response proteins:** CR leads to the elevated expression of heat shock proteins, antioxidant enzymes, and other protective molecules.

- **Improved resilience:** Cells and organisms under CR often show enhanced resistance to oxidative stress, toxins, and other age-associated stressors.
- **Epigenetic orchestration:** The expression of stress response genes is tightly regulated by epigenetic mechanisms, with specific DNA methylation patterns and histone configurations ensuring timely and adequate responses to environmental challenges.

Concluding Thoughts

The molecular pathways influenced by CR paint a picture of a coordinated and multi-faceted response to nutrient scarcity. At the heart of this response lies the epigenome, a dynamic entity that integrates environmental cues to modulate gene expression patterns. As we decipher the intricate dance between CR, molecular pathways, and the epigenome, we inch closer to harnessing the profound benefits of CR, potentially ushering in interventions that can extend healthspan and lifespan.

Implications for Human Diet and Longevity

Caloric restriction (CR) has offered compelling insights into the intricacies of aging and longevity, showing consistent lifespan-extending effects across diverse species. As we navigate the complexities of CR's molecular underpinnings, an equally pressing question arises: What does this mean for human diet and longevity? Can the benefits observed in laboratory organisms be translated to humans? And, if so, how might we incorporate these insights into our dietary habits?

Translating Animal Data to Human Longevity

While CR's benefits are well-documented in animal models, extrapolating these findings to humans is nuanced.

- **Conserved responses:** Many molecular pathways influenced by CR, such as mTOR and sirtuin pathways, are conserved across species, suggesting potential relevance to human health and longevity.

- **Physiological improvements:** Short-term human CR studies have reported better metabolic profiles, reduced inflammation, and improved cardiovascular markers, mirroring observations in animal models.

- **Lifespan extension:** Direct evidence of CR extending human lifespan is, understandably, lacking due to the challenges of long-term controlled studies. However, observations from populations with naturally lower caloric intakes hint at potential longevity benefits.

Epigenetics: Bridging Diet and Lifespan in Humans

Epigenetic markers, especially DNA methylation patterns, offer a promising avenue for understanding CR's effects on human longevity.

- **The epigenetic clock:** DNA methylation patterns can predict biological age, and variations in these patterns, influenced by diet and other factors, might provide insights into an Individual's aging trajectory.

- **Dietary modulation:** Human studies suggest that certain diets can influence epigenetic markers. For instance, diets rich in methyl donors, like folate, can alter DNA methylation patterns.

- **CR's epigenetic influence:** Preliminary human CR studies indicate shifts in DNA methylation patterns, possibly influencing genes associated with aging and age-related diseases.

Practical Implications: Adapting CR for Human Lifestyles

While the concept of reducing caloric intake might sound simple, its practical application in contemporary human societies is riddled with challenges.

- **Intermittent fasting:** Instead of continuous calorie restriction, intermittent fasting (cycles of eating and fasting) might offer similar benefits without the challenges of sustained reduced calorie intake. Studies suggest that intermittent fasting can improve metabolic health and possibly influence longevity-associated epigenetic markers.

- **Dietary quality over quantity:** Rather than merely focusing on calorie count, emphasizing nutrient-dense foods might harness CR's benefits. Diets rich in vegetables, fruits, whole grains, and lean proteins can provide essential nutrients without excessive calories.

- **Personalized approaches:** Genetic and epigenetic variations mean that a one-size-fits-all CR approach is unlikely. Personalized dietary recommendations, based on individual genetic and epigenetic profiles, might be the future of longevity-focused nutrition.

Social and Psychological Dimensions

Implementing CR or CR-mimicking diets isn't just a biological challenge—it's a social and psychological one too.

- **Perceptions of dieting:** The societal obsession with dieting for aesthetic purposes can confound the genuine health benefits of CR. Differentiating between the two is crucial for mental well-being.

- **Cultural considerations:** In many cultures, food plays a central social role. Implementing CR in such contexts requires careful consideration of social norms and practices.

- **Psychological effects:** While CR might offer physiological benefits, its psychological effects, such as potential impacts on mood or cognition, need thorough exploration.

Potential Risks and Considerations

Like any intervention, CR comes with potential risks that need careful consideration.

- **Malnutrition:** Reducing calorie intake without ensuring nutrient adequacy can lead to malnutrition, offsetting any potential longevity benefits.

- **Bone health:** Some studies suggest potential detrimental effects of CR on bone density, warranting caution, especially in populations already at risk for osteoporosis.
- **Fertility implications:** CR can influence reproductive health, possibly impacting fertility. This aspect needs thorough exploration before recommending CR to individuals in their reproductive years.

Concluding Thoughts

Caloric restriction's tale is a testament to the intricate interplay between diet, genes, and the environment. As we look to harness CR's benefits for human health and longevity, a holistic approach is imperative—one that balances biological insights with psychological well-being and societal considerations. While the journey from laboratory benches to dining tables is complex, the promise of healthier, longer lives makes it a pursuit worth every challenge.

Chapter 5:
Histones and Aging

Basics of Histone Modifications

Histones, the protein spools around which our DNA winds, are far more than mere structural entities. These proteins undergo various modifications, determining the accessibility of DNA to transcriptional machinery and influencing gene expression. As such, histone modifications play pivotal roles in numerous biological processes, including those related to aging. Let's delve into the foundational concepts of histone modifications and their implications for the broader epigenetic landscape.

The Structure and Role of Histones

To understand histone modifications, we must first appreciate the structural role of histones in organizing DNA.

- **Nucleosome core:** DNA winds around a histone octamer, consisting of two copies each of histone proteins H2A, H2B, H3, and H4, to form a nucleosome. This arrangement compacts DNA and organizes it within the cell nucleus.

- **Histone H1:** This histone binds to the DNA linking one nucleosome to the next, aiding further compaction.

- **Chromatin states:** Depending on how tightly DNA is wound around histones, chromatin (the combination of DNA and histones) can be in a more open (euchromatin) or closed (heterochromatin) state, influencing gene accessibility and expression.

Types of Histone Modifications

Histones undergo various post-translational modifications, primarily on their protruding N-terminal tails. These modifications serve as epigenetic marks, influencing the chromatin structure and recruitment of other proteins.

- **Acetylation:** The addition of an acetyl group to lysine residues on histone tails, typically associated with gene activation. Acetylation neutralizes the positive charge on lysines, weakening the interaction between histones and the negatively charged DNA, thus allowing for a more open chromatin state.

- **Methylation:** The addition of one, two, or three methyl groups to lysine or arginine residues. Methylation's effects on gene expression are context-dependent, with certain methylation marks being associated with activation and others with repression.

- **Phosphorylation, ubiquitination, and sumoylation:** Beyond acetylation and methylation, histones can undergo other modifications, such as the addition of phosphate, ubiquitin, or small ubiquitin-like modifier (SUMO) groups. Each has specific functional implications for chromatin dynamics and gene expression.

Enzymes Mediating Histone Modifications

Histone modifications are dynamically regulated by enzymes that add or remove these marks.

- **Histone acetyltransferases (HATs):** These enzymes add acetyl groups to histones, promoting gene activation.

- **Histone deacetylases (HDACs):** Opposing the action of HATs, HDACs remove acetyl groups, typically leading to gene repression.

- **Histone methyltransferases (HMTs):** These enzymes methylate lysine or arginine residues on histones. Depending on the specific residue and degree of methylation, this can either activate or repress gene expression.

- **Histone demethylases:** These enzymes remove methyl groups, counteracting the effects of HMTs.

Histone Modifications and Gene Regulation

The orchestration of histone modifications influences the epigenetic landscape and, consequently, gene expression.

- **Reading the histone code:** Specific patterns of histone modifications, often termed the "histone code," can recruit or repel various proteins. For instance, certain marks attract transcriptional activators, while others attract repressors.

- **Synergy and antagonism:** Some histone modifications can co-exist and synergize to fine-tune gene expression, while others are mutually exclusive or antagonistic.

- **Cross-talk with DNA methylation:** Histone modifications often intersect with DNA methylation patterns. For instance, certain histone marks are associated with DNA methylation, reinforcing gene repression.

Implications for Cellular Memory and Identity

The patterns of histone modifications contribute to the cellular memory, ensuring genes appropriate for a specific cell type are expressed while others are repressed.

- **Stable marks:** Some histone modifications are stably maintained and can be passed on during cell division, preserving cellular identity.

- **Dynamic changes:** In contrast, other modifications are more dynamic, responding to environmental cues or cellular signals, allowing cells to adapt and modify gene expression accordingly.

Concluding Thoughts

Histone modifications offer a rich layer of regulation over our genetic blueprint. These marks, in their intricate patterns, determine which genes are expressed, when, and to what extent. As we will see in subsequent sections, the changes in these modifications, particularly in the context of aging, can have profound effects on cellular function, healthspan, and longevity.

The Role of Histones in Gene Expression

At the heart of cellular functionality is the fundamental process of gene expression, where the information coded within DNA is transcribed into RNA and then often translated into proteins. Playing a central role in this process are histones, around which DNA is wound. Far from being passive DNA spools, histones actively influence which genes are accessible for transcription. Let's delve deeper into how histones govern gene expression and, by extension, cell fate and function.

The Fundamental Unit: The Nucleosome

Understanding the role of histones begins with the nucleosome.

- **Nucleosome structure:** Each nucleosome comprises approximately 147 base pairs of DNA wrapped around a histone octamer. This octamer includes two each of H2A, H2B, H3, and H4 histone proteins.

- **Barrier to transcription:** With DNA wound around histones, the transcriptional machinery cannot readily access it. Thus, nucleosome positioning and modifications can either permit or prevent gene transcription.

Chromatin Remodeling and Accessibility

The DNA-histone structure is not static. Chromatin remodelers adjust nucleosome positions, thereby affecting gene accessibility.

- **Sliding:** Chromatin remodeling complexes can slide nucleosomes along the DNA, revealing or concealing specific DNA regions.

- **Ejection and replacement:** Remodelers can also temporarily eject histones, allowing transcription factors and other machinery to access the DNA.

- **Incorporation of histone variants:** Histone variants, which have slightly different structures than canonical histones, can be incorporated into nucleosomes. These variants can influence gene expression by altering nucleosome stability or by creating unique surfaces for protein interactions.

The Epigenetic Language of Histone Modifications

As previously discussed, histones can undergo various post-translational modifications. These modifications play instrumental roles in dictating gene expression patterns.

- **Active marks:** Some histone modifications, such as the acetylation of certain lysine residues, generally mark regions of active transcription. These marks create a more open chromatin structure and can recruit proteins that facilitate transcription.

- **Repressive marks:** In contrast, other modifications, like specific methylation marks, are associated with gene silencing. These marks often lead to compact chromatin structures that are less accessible to transcriptional machinery.

- **Combination codes:** Often, multiple modifications coexist on the same histone tail, creating a combination or "code." This histone code can recruit specific protein complexes that determine the transcriptional status of a given gene.

Histone Modifiers and Readers

The enzymes that add or remove histone modifications, as well as the proteins that "read" these marks, play critical roles in gene regulation.

- **Writers:** Enzymes like histone acetyltransferases (HATs) and histone methyltransferases (HMTs) add modifications to histones, influencing chromatin structure and gene activity.

- **Erasers:** On the other hand, enzymes like histone deacetylases (HDACs) and histone demethylases remove these marks, allowing for dynamic regulation of gene expression.

- **Readers:** Certain proteins have domains that recognize and bind specific histone modifications. Once bound, these proteins can recruit other factors that activate or repress transcription or further modify chromatin structure.

Histones and Aging: A Dynamic Interplay

The pattern of histone modifications is not static throughout an organism's life. Changes in these patterns can influence the aging process.

- **Loss of marks:** With age, there can be a global loss of certain histone marks, leading to changes in gene expression patterns.
- **Positional changes:** Aging can also lead to the relocation of nucleosomes, affecting which genes are accessible for transcription.
- **Aging and cellular stress:** Cellular stresses, which accumulate with age, can induce specific histone modifications. These marks can activate stress response genes or promote DNA repair.
- **Histone variants:** The incorporation of histone variants can change with age, influencing chromatin structure and gene expression in aging cells.

Concluding Reflections

Histones play a central role in the orchestration of gene expression. By modulating the accessibility of DNA and recruiting specific protein complexes, histones ensure that genes are expressed in the right cells at the right times. As organisms age, changes in histone modifications and positioning can have profound effects on cellular function and, by extension, on healthspan and longevity. Understanding these dynamic processes offers potential avenues for interventions that can modulate the aging trajectory and promote healthy aging.

How Aging Influences and Is Influenced by Histone Modifications

Aging, an inescapable biological phenomenon, is shaped by a plethora of genetic and environmental factors. At the molecular level, changes in histone modifications play a pivotal role in the aging process, influencing gene expression, genome stability, and cellular function. This intricate dance between aging and histone modifications offers insights into the progression of aging and reveals potential avenues for therapeutic interventions.

Global Loss of Histone Proteins and Modifications

As an organism ages, the chromatin landscape undergoes significant alterations. One such change is the global reduction in core histone protein levels.

- **Histone reduction:** Studies have demonstrated a decrease in histones H3 and H4 in aged yeast, worms, and flies. In mammals, aging-associated histone loss has been observed in specific tissues.
- **Implications:** Reduced histone levels can lead to a more relaxed chromatin structure, which can, in turn, affect gene expression, genome stability, and DNA repair mechanisms.

Changes in Specific Histone Modifications

Aging does not only lead to a decline in total histone amounts but also induces changes in specific histone modifications.

- **Repressive marks:** With age, there is an accumulation of certain repressive histone marks, like H3K9me3 and H3K27me3, in various organisms. This increase in repressive marks can lead to silencing of genes critical for youthful cellular function.
- **Active marks:** Conversely, some active marks, like H4K16 acetylation, decrease with age. This reduction can result in the repression of genes required for proper cellular activities.

The Role of Sirtuins: From Histones to Aging

Sirtuins, a family of NAD+-dependent protein deacetylases, are intimately linked with aging and histone modifications.

- **Deacetylation:** Sirtuins, particularly SIRT1 in mammals, remove acetyl groups from specific lysine residues on histones, influencing chromatin compaction and gene expression.

- **Lifespan extension:** In various organisms, from yeast to mammals, sirtuin activation or overexpression has been linked to lifespan extension. This longevity effect is, in part, attributed to sirtuins' role in histone deacetylation and consequent gene regulation.

- **Caloric restriction:** One of the most consistent lifespan-extending interventions, caloric restriction, elevates NAD+ levels, enhancing sirtuin activity. This elevated sirtuin activity leads to changes in histone acetylation patterns, affecting the expression of longevity-associated genes.

Histone Modifications and DNA Damage Response

With age, cells accumulate DNA damage. Histone modifications play a crucial role in the DNA damage response, ensuring genome integrity.

- **Recognition and signaling:** When DNA damage occurs, specific histone modifications are added around the damage site. For instance, the phosphorylation of H2AX (yielding γH2AX) is a marker for DNA double-strand breaks.

- **Recruitment of repair machinery:** These damage-associated histone marks help recruit DNA repair proteins to the lesion site, facilitating efficient and accurate repair.

- **Impaired response in aging:** As organisms age, the efficiency of this histone modification-mediated DNA damage response can decline, leading to increased genomic instability, a hallmark of aging.

Changes in Histone Variants with Age

In addition to canonical histones, special histone variants can replace standard histones in certain nucleosomes. Aging influences the distribution and incorporation of these variants.

- **H3.3 variant:** In mammals, H3.3 is a replacement variant that gets incorporated outside of DNA replication. Studies indicate altered distribution of H3.3 in aged cells, influencing gene expression patterns.

- **MacroH2A:** This is another histone variant that accumulates in certain aged tissues. Its incorporation has implications for chromatin structure and gene regulation.

Histone Modifications in Age-related Diseases

Many age-related diseases, such as neurodegenerative disorders and cancers, have been associated with changes in histone modifications.

- **Alzheimer's disease:** In the brains of Alzheimer's patients, there are altered patterns of histone acetylation and methylation, which can influence the expression of genes related to neuronal function and survival.
- **Cancer:** The transformation of a normal cell to a cancerous one often involves changes in histone modifications. For instance, globally reduced levels of H4K16 acetylation and H4K20 methylation are hallmarks of many cancer types.

Concluding Insights

The intricate interplay between histone modifications and aging shapes the trajectory of an organism's life. These epigenetic alterations influence gene expression, genome stability, and cellular responses to stress. By understanding these dynamics, researchers hope to unveil therapeutic targets to mitigate age-associated decline and extend healthspan. Indeed, the epigenetic landscape offers a promising frontier in the quest to comprehend and modulate aging.

Chapter 6: Transgenerational Epigenetic Inheritance

The Debate over Inheritance of Acquired Traits

The idea that organisms can pass on characteristics acquired during their lifetimes to their offspring has been a topic of debate for centuries. Stemming from early speculations by Jean-Baptiste Lamarck, this concept contrasts with the Mendelian understanding of inheritance, where genes remain unaltered by environmental influences. The emergent field of transgenerational epigenetic inheritance has reignited this debate, challenging traditional paradigms and offering new insights Into how life experiences can shape subsequent generations.

Jean-Baptiste Lamarck and the Legacy of Lamarckism

To grasp the modern debate, it's crucial to understand its historical origins.

- **Lamarck's theory:** In the early 19th century, Lamarck proposed that organisms could alter their traits in response to their environment and then pass on these acquired characteristics to their offspring. For instance, he speculated that giraffes developed long necks by stretching to reach high foliage, and then passed this trait on.

- **The decline of Lamarckism:** With the advent of Mendelian genetics and Darwinian evolution in the late 19th and early 20th centuries, Lamarck's ideas largely fell out of favor. It became accepted that DNA sequences were stable across generations, unaffected by external influences.

Modern Epigenetics and the Revival of Lamarckian Ideas

With advances in molecular biology and the discovery of mechanisms that can modify gene expression without altering DNA sequence, Lamarckian ideas experienced a revival.

- **Epigenetic markers:** These are chemical modifications on DNA or histone proteins that can change gene expression patterns. Importantly, some of these markers can be influenced by environmental factors, such as diet, toxins, or stress.

- **Transgenerational inheritance:** In certain cases, these epigenetic changes can be passed on to subsequent generations, even if those generations aren't directly exposed to the initial environmental trigger.

Experimental Evidence and Notable Cases

Several studies have provided evidence supporting transgenerational epigenetic inheritance.

- **The Agouti mouse:** A classic example involves the Agouti mouse, where a particular epigenetic mark can lead to yellow fur and obesity. When pregnant mice are exposed to certain dietary supplements, the epigenetic marks change, leading to offspring with brown fur and normal weight. Importantly, these changes can persist in subsequent generations.

- **Famine and human health:** In humans, historical events like the Dutch Hunger Winter during World War II have indicated potential transgenerational effects. Descendants of individuals who experienced the famine during pregnancy show altered health outcomes, suggesting possible epigenetic inheritance.

Skepticism and Challenges

While there is growing evidence for transgenerational epigenetic inheritance, the concept remains controversial for several reasons.

- **Mechanistic uncertainties:** The exact mechanisms underlying epigenetic inheritance are not fully understood. During

reproduction, most epigenetic marks are erased and reset, so
how certain marks escape this reset remains a question.

- **Limited examples:** While some compelling cases exist, there
  are relatively few well-documented instances of transgenerational epigenetic inheritance, especially in humans.

- **Genetic confounders:** Some argue that observed transgenerational effects may arise from traditional genetic inheritance
  or from shared environmental factors across generations,
  rather than from epigenetic mechanisms.

Implications for Evolutionary Biology

If transgenerational epigenetic inheritance occurs regularly, it
could have profound implications for our understanding of evolution.

- **Rapid adaptation:** Epigenetic changes can occur rapidly in
  response to environmental shifts, potentially allowing populations to adapt quicker than through traditional genetic
  evolution.

- **Evolutionary 'memory':** Epigenetic markers could provide a
  sort of 'memory' of past environmental conditions, inform-
  ing the development and survival strategies of subsequent
  generations.

- **Interplay with traditional genetics:** Some propose that epigenetic changes might guide subsequent genetic changes,
  acting as a precursor to more stable genetic adaptations.

Conclusion: An Evolving Understanding

While the debate over the inheritance of acquired traits is far from
settled, it's clear that the traditional Mendelian view of inheritance
is only part of the story. Transgenerational epigenetic inheritance
challenges long-held beliefs, prompting scientists to rethink how
organisms adapt and evolve. As research progresses, we will likely
develop a more nuanced understanding of inheritance, where
both genetic and epigenetic factors interplay to shape the trajectories of lineages across generations.

Studies Supporting Epigenetic Inheritance Across Generations

Transgenerational epigenetic inheritance has generated considerable interest and debate in the scientific community. While traditional genetics emphasizes the stability of DNA across generations, research into epigenetic inheritance explores how life experiences and environmental factors might cause inheritable changes in gene expression without altering DNA sequences. Numerous studies across different organisms have delved into this concept, offering compelling evidence for the existence of such non-DNA-sequence-based inheritance.

The Agouti Mouse: A Colorful Tale of Epigenetics

One of the most cited examples of epigenetic inheritance involves the Agouti viable yellow (A^vy) mouse.

- **Phenotype variation:** The A^vy allele causes variation in coat color in mice, ranging from yellow to mottled to brown. Interestingly, this variation doesn't arise from DNA mutations but from epigenetic differences, specifically DNA methylation.

- **Dietary influence:** When pregnant mice carrying the A^vy allele are fed a diet rich in methyl donors, such as folic acid or choline, the offspring tend to have more of the brown phenotype due to increased methylation.

- **Transgenerational effects:** This dietary intervention doesn't just affect the immediate offspring. Subsequent generations, even without direct dietary exposure, also exhibit increased brown coat prevalence, suggesting a transgenerational epigenetic inheritance.

Vinclozolin and Reproductive Changes in Rats

A landmark study on the fungicide vinclozolin revealed startling transgenerational effects on rat reproduction.

- **Direct exposure:** Male rats exposed to vinclozolin during embryonic development exhibited reduced sperm quality and increased infertility.

- **Transgenerational repercussions:** Astonishingly, these reproductive issues persisted for at least four subsequent generations, even without further direct exposure to the chemical. The proposed mechanism is epigenetic changes in the sperm DNA, which then perpetuate across generations.

Honeybees: A Story of Nutrition and Destiny

The differentiation between queen and worker bees provides a fascinating example of how nutrition influences epigenetic markers and fate.

- **Royal jelly and destiny:** Larvae fed royal jelly develop into queens, while those fed a regular diet become workers. This nutritional difference causes distinct epigenetic patterns, particularly histone modifications.
- **Inheritance of traits:** Recent research suggests that some of these epigenetic marks might be inheritable, influencing the behavior and physiology of subsequent generations.

The Swedish Overkalix Study: Famine's Echo Across Generations

Human studies, though inherently more complex, also hint at the potential for transgenerational epigenetic inheritance.

- **Historical context:** In the 19th century, the Swedish town of Overkalix experienced dramatic fluctuations in food availability due to varying harvests.
- **Generational effects:** By studying historical records and the health outcomes of subsequent generations, researchers found that grandsons of men who experienced abundance during their pre-puberty had a higher risk of dying from diabetes. Conversely, grandsons of men who faced famine during this period lived longer on average.
- **Proposed mechanisms:** While direct evidence of epigenetic modifications was not available, the patterns strongly suggest potential epigenetic changes in sperm cells, influenced by nutrition, that could then affect later generations.

Caenorhabditis elegans and Small RNAs

The nematode worm, C. elegans, offers a compelling model for studying epigenetic inheritance, particularly involving small RNAs.

- **RNA inheritance:** Researchers exposed worms to specific environmental conditions, leading to the production of small RNAs. These molecules, which regulate gene expression, were found in subsequent generations, even those not directly exposed to the initial conditions.

- **Trait persistence:** The phenotypic changes mediated by these small RNAs persisted for multiple generations, showcasing a mechanism by which experiences can influence offspring without changes to DNA sequence.

Contemplations and Considerations

It's essential to approach the topic of transgenerational epigenetic inheritance with caution and rigor. Many of the above studies, though compelling, face challenges such as:

- **Resetting during reproduction:** Most epigenetic marks are reset during the formation of gametes and early embryonic development. How certain epigenetic changes evade this reset is still a topic of active research.

- **Environmental consistency:** Ensuring that observed transgenerational effects aren't due to shared environmental factors, rather than genuine epigenetic inheritance, can be challenging, especially in human studies.

Conclusion: A Dynamic Field with Growing Evidence

Transgenerational epigenetic inheritance remains a frontier in genetic research. While challenges persist, the growing body of evidence from diverse organisms suggests that our understanding of inheritance must expand beyond just DNA sequences. The experiences and environments of ancestors might echo in the genes, physiology, and health of descendants in ways previously unimagined.

Implications for Familial Health and Longevity

The discovery of transgenerational epigenetic inheritance offers a more intricate understanding of the genetic tapestry that determines an individual's health and longevity. The realization that environmental factors and life choices can influence not just one's own health but also that of subsequent generations opens up new avenues for disease prediction, intervention, and understanding family health patterns.

The Shadow of Ancestral Environments

Our ancestors' environments, choices, and experiences can cast a long shadow on our own lives, a notion that resonates deeply with the study of transgenerational epigenetics.

- **Historical events and health outcomes:** As noted in studies like the Swedish Overkalix investigation, the food abundance or scarcity faced by one generation can influence disease risk and life span several generations down the line. Such findings raise the possibility that other large-scale events, such as wars, economic depressions, or pandemics, might also have long-term epigenetic consequences.

- **Predicting familial disease risk:** If a family shows a pattern of a particular health issue, it might not just be traditional genetics at play. Epigenetic inheritance could provide another layer of explanation, broadening our understanding of hereditary disease risk.

Beyond Genetic Counseling: Epigenetic Counseling?

Genetic counseling is a well-established field that assists individuals and families in understanding inherited conditions and their potential risks.

- **Incorporating epigenetics:** With the growing understanding of transgenerational epigenetic inheritance, there's a compelling argument to be made for incorporating epigenetic considerations into such counseling sessions.

- **Holistic family histories:** A more comprehensive approach to family health history would not only consider diseases and conditions but also significant events, exposures, or lifestyle choices that might have epigenetic ramifications.

Health Interventions: A Multi-Generational Perspective

The realization that today's choices can influence the health of descendants offers a powerful incentive for health interventions.

- **Dietary choices:** If a certain diet or exposure can influence not only individual health but also the health of future generations, public health campaigns might stress the multi-generational impact of nutritional choices.

- **Chemical exposures:** Consideration for transgenerational epigenetic effects could influence regulations around chemical exposures, emphasizing not just individual safety but also potential impacts on subsequent generations.

Psychological and Societal Implications

The concept of transgenerational epigenetic inheritance introduces new layers of psychological and societal complexity.

- **Parental responsibility:** The idea that one's actions can directly impact the health and well-being of unborn generations might weigh heavily on individuals, introducing new dimensions of parental or even grandparental responsibility.

- **Societal pressure:** On a societal level, there could be increased pressure or even judgment around lifestyle choices, especially those that might have perceived multi-generational impacts.

Ethical Considerations

Like any advance in genetic understanding, the discovery of transgenerational epigenetic inheritance brings with it a suite of ethical concerns.

- **Privacy:** As we gather more epigenetic data, questions arise about who has access to this information and how it can be used. For instance, could insurers use such data to assess risk?
- **Interventions:** If we develop ways to modify epigenetic marks, should we? What are the ethical implications of altering epigenetic information, especially when its impacts could span generations?

The Evolutionary Perspective: Adapting Across Generations

From an evolutionary standpoint, transgenerational epigenetic inheritance offers a mechanism for populations to rapidly adapt to changing environments.

- **Rapid response to environment:** Unlike genetic mutations, which can take many generations to confer a significant evolutionary advantage, epigenetic changes can occur within a single generation, allowing for quicker adaptation to new challenges or opportunities.
- **Memory of past environments:** Epigenetic marks can serve as a record or memory of past environmental conditions, potentially prepping subsequent generations for similar challenges.

Conclusion: A New Frontier in Family Health and Longevity

Transgenerational epigenetic inheritance, though still a developing field, offers profound insights into human health and longevity. The choices and experiences of ancestors, echoing through epigenetic modifications, underscore the deep interconnectedness of generations. As we continue to unravel these connections, we'll likely find new ways to promote health, prevent disease, and appreciate the myriad factors that determine our familial legacies of health and longevity.

Chapter 7: Epigenetics and Age-Related Diseases

Overview of Common Age-Related Diseases

Age is the most significant risk factor for a myriad of diseases and disorders. As we grow older, our bodies undergo various biological changes that can increase vulnerability to certain conditions. Epigenetic alterations, as they accumulate over time, play a pivotal role in the aging process and, by extension, the onset of age-related diseases. This chapter offers an overview of some common age-related diseases, shedding light on how they manifest and the potential role of epigenetics in their development.

Cardiovascular Diseases (CVDs)

Cardiovascular diseases encompass a range of conditions affecting the heart and blood vessels, including coronary artery disease, heart failure, and stroke.

- **Manifestation:** Symptoms can range from chest pain (angina) to shortness of breath, fatigue, or even sudden cardiac events.

- **Epigenetic considerations:** DNA methylation patterns and histone modifications have been observed in atherosclerotic lesions. Alterations in these epigenetic marks may influence gene expression patterns related to inflammation, lipid metabolism, and plaque stability.

Alzheimer's Disease and Other Dementias

Alzheimer's disease is a progressive neurodegenerative condition, leading to severe cognitive impairment. It represents the majority of dementia cases.

- **Manifestation:** Initial symptoms often include forgetfulness or difficulty in performing familiar tasks, progressing to severe memory loss, confusion, and behavioral changes.

- **Epigenetic considerations:** Epigenetic changes, such as altered DNA methylation patterns, have been identified in the brains of Alzheimer's patients. These changes may impact genes crucial for synaptic plasticity and neuronal health.

Osteoporosis

Osteoporosis is a skeletal disorder characterized by compromised bone strength, predisposing individuals to increased fracture risk.

- **Manifestation:** Often asymptomatic until a fracture occurs, common fracture sites include the hip, spine, and wrist.

- **Epigenetic considerations:** DNA methylation and histone modification patterns in bone cells can influence bone density. Alterations in these patterns might play a role in the pathogenesis of osteoporosis.

Type 2 Diabetes Mellitus (T2DM)

Type 2 diabetes is characterized by resistance to insulin or inadequate insulin production, leading to elevated blood sugar levels.

- **Manifestation:** Symptoms include excessive thirst, frequent urination, fatigue, blurred vision, and slow wound healing.

- **Epigenetic considerations:** Epigenetic changes in genes related to insulin signaling, glucose metabolism, and pancreatic beta-cell function have been implicated in T2DM onset and progression.

Age-Related Macular Degeneration (AMD)

AMD affects the central region of the retina (macula), leading to vision loss primarily in the center field of vision.

- **Manifestation:** Blurred or no vision in the center visual field, often starting as a dark, blurry area.
- **Epigenetic considerations:** Epigenetic regulation of genes involved in retinal health, inflammation, and angiogenesis can play a role in the onset and progression of AMD.

Parkinson's Disease

Parkinson's is a neurodegenerative disorder affecting motor function due to the loss of dopamine-producing brain cells.

- **Manifestation:** Symptoms start gradually, often with a slight tremor in one hand. Other symptoms include slowed movement, muscle rigidity, and impaired posture.
- **Epigenetic considerations:** Changes in DNA methylation patterns and histone modifications in genes associated with neuronal health and dopamine production have been observed in Parkinson's patients.

Rheumatoid Arthritis

Rheumatoid arthritis is an autoimmune disease wherein the immune system attacks the synovium — the lining of the membranes surrounding the joints.

- **Manifestation:** Joint pain, swelling, stiffness, and over time, joint damage and deformation.
- **Epigenetic considerations:** Epigenetic modifications in immune cells can impact gene expression patterns related to inflammation, leading to joint damage.

Conclusion: A Complex Interplay Between Age and Disease

The above diseases highlight the multifaceted nature of age-related conditions, with each having its unique set of genetic and environmental risk factors. As research advances, the role of epigenetics in these diseases becomes increasingly apparent. Understanding these epigenetic changes offers not only insights into disease mechanisms but also potential avenues for intervention, diagnosis, and personalized treatments. As we continue to explore the complexities of age-related diseases, the intertwining of genetics, epigenetics, and environmental factors will undoubtedly remain central to our comprehension and management of these conditions.

The Role of Epigenetic Changes in Disease Onset and Progression

Epigenetics, the study of heritable changes in gene function that don't involve alterations to the underlying DNA sequence, plays a crucial role in various biological processes, including cellular differentiation, development, and response to environmental stimuli. Significantly, epigenetic alterations have been implicated in the onset and progression of numerous diseases, especially age-related ones. Understanding how these changes contribute to disease can offer insights into its prevention, diagnosis, and treatment.

How Epigenetic Changes Occur

Epigenetic changes primarily encompass DNA methylation, histone modifications, and non-coding RNA interactions. These modifications can be influenced by various factors, including:

- **Environmental stimuli:** Factors such as diet, stress, and exposure to toxins can induce epigenetic changes, potentially leading to disease states.

- **Aging:** As one ages, the epigenome undergoes shifts that can influence gene expression patterns, contributing to age-associated diseases.

- **Genetic predisposition:** Genetic variations can predispose individuals to certain epigenetic alterations, heightening their risk for specific diseases.

Epigenetic Changes in Cancer

Cancer is a prime example of how epigenetic alterations can drive disease. Changes in DNA methylation patterns and histone modifications can result in:

- **Gene silencing:** Tumor suppressor genes can be silenced through hypermethylation, reducing their ability to prevent uncontrolled cell growth.
- **Activation of oncogenes:** On the other hand, oncogenes, which promote cell growth and proliferation, might become overactive due to hypomethylation.

Cardiovascular Diseases and Epigenetics

Cardiovascular diseases (CVDs), which remain leading causes of death worldwide, have been linked to epigenetic changes, particularly DNA methylation patterns that influence:

- **Endothelial function:** Epigenetic modifications can impact genes crucial for maintaining the integrity and function of blood vessel walls.
- **Lipid metabolism:** Alterations in the epigenome can affect lipid metabolism, leading to atherosclerosis, a condition where fatty deposits narrow and block arteries.

Neurodegenerative Diseases

Conditions like Alzheimer's and Parkinson's diseases see significant epigenetic involvement. For instance:

- **Alzheimer's disease:** Aberrant DNA methylation and histone acetylation patterns can impact genes essential for synaptic function, memory formation, and neural plasticity.
- **Parkinson's disease:** Epigenetic changes in genes associated with dopamine production can affect motor function and cognition.

Diabetes Mellitus

Type 2 diabetes, characterized by insulin resistance, has been associated with epigenetic changes affecting:

- **Insulin signaling:** Modifications in the epigenome can influence insulin receptor expression and downstream signaling pathways.
- **Beta-cell function:** Epigenetic alterations can affect the function and survival of insulin-producing beta cells in the pancreas.

Autoimmune Disorders

Conditions like rheumatoid arthritis and lupus, where the body's immune system mistakenly attacks its tissues, are influenced by epigenetic changes that:

- **Alter immune cell differentiation:** Epigenetic modifications can skew the differentiation of immune cells, leading to enhanced inflammatory responses.
- **Impact cytokine production:** Cytokines are signaling molecules crucial for immune responses. Epigenetic changes can affect their production, exacerbating disease symptoms.

Epigenetics and Disease Progression

Beyond disease onset, epigenetic changes play a significant role in disease progression and severity. For example:

- **Cancer metastasis:** Epigenetic alterations can activate genes that promote cancer cell migration and invasion, leading to metastasis or the spread of cancer to other parts of the body.
- **Progression of neurodegeneration:** In conditions like Alzheimer's, accumulating epigenetic changes can exacerbate neuronal loss, speeding up cognitive decline.

Epigenetic Markers as Diagnostic Tools

Given their significance in disease onset and progression, epigenetic markers are emerging as potential diagnostic tools:

- **Early detection:** Changes in DNA methylation patterns can serve as early indicators for conditions like cancer, even before the manifestation of clear clinical symptoms.
- **Disease prognosis:** Epigenetic markers can offer insights into disease severity and potential progression, aiding in patient management.

Therapeutic Implications

Understanding epigenetic changes in diseases opens doors for novel therapeutic interventions:

- **Epigenetic drugs:** Compounds that can modify epigenetic marks, such as DNA methyltransferase inhibitors or histone deacetylase inhibitors, offer potential treatment avenues, especially in cancers.
- **Personalized medicine:** Epigenetic profiling can guide treatment decisions, allowing for tailored therapies that address individual epigenomic landscapes.

Conclusion: A Deeper Understanding of Disease

The nexus between epigenetics and disease offers a more nuanced understanding of pathogenesis. As we continue to unravel the intricate tapestry of the epigenome and its influence on health and disease, there's hope for improved diagnostics, treatments, and perhaps even preventive measures that target the very core of gene regulation.

Potential for Epigenetic Therapies

In the ever-evolving field of medicine, epigenetic therapies have emerged as a beacon of hope for treating age-related diseases and potentially rejuvenating biological processes. Unlike traditional genetic therapies, which aim to replace or correct mutated genes, epigenetic therapies target the molecular tags that influence gene expression without changing the DNA sequence. Given the increasing understanding of the role epigenetics plays in age-related diseases, harnessing the power of these therapies could revolutionize medicine.

Epigenetic Dysregulation and Disease

Before delving into the potential of epigenetic therapies, it's pivotal to understand how epigenetic dysregulation contributes to disease. From cancers to neurodegenerative disorders, aberrant patterns of DNA methylation, histone modifications, and non-coding RNA interactions can disrupt normal cellular functions:

- **Promotion of oncogenes:** In cancer, aberrant hypomethylation can activate oncogenes, fueling tumor growth.

- **Silencing of tumor suppressor genes:** Conversely, hypermethylation can silence tumor suppressor genes, removing barriers to uncontrolled cell proliferation.

- **Impaired neural plasticity:** In neurodegenerative diseases, altered histone acetylation patterns can inhibit genes essential for synaptic function, impeding neural plasticity and memory formation.

Current Epigenetic Therapies in Use

Several epigenetic drugs have already been approved for clinical use, mainly for hematologic malignancies:

- **DNA methyltransferase inhibitors (DNMTi):** Drugs like azacitidine and decitabine inhibit the addition of methyl groups to DNA. They've been approved for the treatment of myelodysplastic syndromes, acting by reactivating silenced tumor suppressor genes.

- **Histone deacetylase inhibitors (HDACi):** Vorinostat and romidepsin inhibit enzymes responsible for removing acetyl groups from histones. They're used to treat cutaneous T-cell lymphoma, with their primary mechanism being the reactivation of silenced genes that regulate cell growth.

Potential Applications of Epigenetic Therapies

Beyond existing treatments, research is uncovering potential applications for epigenetic therapies in a broad spectrum of diseases:

- **Neurodegenerative diseases:** Therapies that modulate histone acetylation, methylation, or non-coding RNA interactions have shown promise in preclinical models of diseases like Alzheimer's and Parkinson's. By reactivating genes that promote neural plasticity and synaptic function, these therapies could potentially slow or reverse disease progression.

- **Autoimmune disorders:** Epigenetic drugs can potentially recalibrate the immune system, modulating the differentiation of immune cells and reducing inflammatory responses typical in autoimmune diseases.

- **Age-related macular degeneration (AMD):** Preliminary research has suggested that epigenetic modifications play a role in AMD, implying that epigenetic therapies might help preserve vision in affected individuals.

Rejuvenation and Age Reversal

One of the most tantalizing prospects of epigenetic therapies is their potential role in biological rejuvenation:

- **Targeting the epigenetic clock:** As we age, specific patterns of DNA methylation accumulate, serving as markers of biological age. By targeting these patterns, epigenetic therapies could potentially "turn back the clock," making cells functionally younger.

- **Stem cell rejuvenation:** Aging stem cells lose their ability to differentiate into various cell types. Epigenetic therapies might rejuvenate these cells, enhancing tissue repair and regeneration.

Challenges in Epigenetic Therapies

Despite their potential, several challenges need to be addressed:

- **Specificity:** The epigenome is vast and complex. Targeting one epigenetic mark might inadvertently affect others, leading to off-target effects.
- **Delivery:** Efficiently delivering epigenetic drugs to the right cells or tissues remains a challenge. Some current methods might not be suitable for all diseases or might carry side effects.
- **Long-term effects:** The long-term effects of epigenetic modulation remain largely unknown. For instance, reactivating a silenced tumor suppressor gene might benefit cancer patients, but if other genes are unsilenced simultaneously, new health issues could arise.

Future Directions

With rapid advancements in technology and our understanding of the epigenome:

- **Personalized epigenetic treatments:** As with other areas of medicine, there's a push towards personalized treatments. By mapping an individual's epigenome, therapies can be tailored for maximum benefit and minimal side effects.
- **Combination therapies:** Combining epigenetic drugs with other treatments, such as traditional chemotherapy in cancer, might enhance efficacy.
- **Biomarker discovery:** As the field matures, discovering new epigenetic markers for disease diagnosis, prognosis, and therapeutic response will be pivotal.

Conclusion: A New Horizon in Medicine

Epigenetic therapies hold the promise of a paradigm shift in how we approach age-related diseases and aging itself. By targeting the molecular mechanisms that regulate gene expression, these treatments could offer solutions where traditional genetics-based therapies fall short. As research continues and the potential of epigenetic therapies becomes clearer, we stand on the cusp of a new era in medicine.

Chapter 8: Reversing the Clock – The Future of Epigenetic Therapies

Current State of Research on Epigenetic Rejuvenation

Epigenetic rejuvenation is a burgeoning frontier in the realms of biology and medicine. At its core, it seeks to reverse or mitigate the epigenetic changes that accompany aging, effectively rejuvenating cells and tissues to a more youthful state. As our understanding of the intricate dance between genetics, epigenetics, and aging deepens, researchers are striving to harness epigenetic modifications to reverse cellular age, repair damage, and combat age-related diseases. This chapter delves into the latest insights and breakthroughs in the realm of epigenetic rejuvenation.

Epigenetic Clocks and Their Significance

Central to the quest for rejuvenation is the understanding of the "epigenetic clock". This clock is a collection of DNA methylation sites that predict chronological age with astonishing accuracy. Researchers like Dr. Steve Horvath have refined algorithms that, by analyzing the methylation status of specific genomic sites, can estimate the biological age of a tissue, cell type, or even the entire organism.

The divergence between biological and chronological age can serve as an indicator of health and potential longevity. Individuals whose biological age is greater than their chronological age often show early signs of age-related diseases.

Key Breakthroughs in Epigenetic Rejuvenation

Several groundbreaking studies have demonstrated the potential of epigenetic interventions to reverse aspects of aging:

- **Yamanaka Factors:** In 2006, Dr. Shinya Yamanaka identified a set of four transcription factors that can revert mature cells to a pluripotent stem cell state. Later experiments indicated that transient exposure to these Yamanaka factors could reverse signs of aging in cells and tissues without inducing pluripotency, highlighting a potential avenue for rejuvenation.

- **Targeted Epigenetic Reversion:** Leveraging CRISPR technology, researchers have selectively targeted and modulated specific epigenetic sites associated with aging. Such targeted reversion holds promise for precision rejuvenation without the unintended consequences of broad epigenetic modulation.

- **Dietary and Pharmacological Interventions:** Certain compounds, like resveratrol (found in grapes) and metformin (a diabetes drug), have demonstrated potential in modulating epigenetic markers and extending lifespan in animal models.

Challenges in Translating Research to Therapies

While the promise of epigenetic rejuvenation is tantalizing, several hurdles need to be overcome:

- **Safety Concerns:** Overzealous reversion might induce cells to become pluripotent or transform into cancerous cells. Striking the right balance between rejuvenation and safety is crucial.

- **Tissue Specificity:** Epigenetic landscapes vary across tissues. A therapeutic intervention that works for one tissue type might not be effective, or even safe, for another.

- **Long-Term Implications:** The long-term effects of epigenetic rejuvenation are not fully understood. Rejuvenated cells might have different functional properties, or there might be unforeseen consequences that manifest over time.

The Road Ahead: Next Steps in Epigenetic Rejuvenation

The realm of epigenetic rejuvenation is ripe for exploration, and several avenues are emerging as particularly promising:

- **Personalized Rejuvenation Protocols:** As our understanding of individual epigenomes deepens, it might become possible to develop personalized rejuvenation strategies tailored to an individual's unique epigenetic landscape.
- **Combination Therapies:** Combining epigenetic interventions with other age-reversing strategies, like senolytics (drugs that target senescent cells), might produce synergistic effects.
- **Biomarker Development:** Refining and expanding our repertoire of epigenetic aging biomarkers can provide more precise tools for gauging rejuvenation efficacy and monitoring potential side effects.

Conclusion: The Dawn of a New Era

The current state of research in epigenetic rejuvenation is at an exciting juncture. The interplay between aging and epigenetics is intricate, and while many pieces of the puzzle remain to be placed, the picture that's emerging is one of immense promise. We're beginning to unlock the secrets of the epigenome and its role in aging, paving the way for interventions that might one day reverse the clock on cellular aging.

While challenges and uncertainties lie ahead, the potential rewards — extended healthspan, mitigation of age-related diseases, and perhaps even a degree of biological immortality — drive researchers and clinicians forward in this thrilling odyssey.

The Potential and Challenges of Age-Reversal Therapies

The concept of age-reversal, once a domain relegated to the pages of science fiction, has taken root in scientific communities across the world. As our understanding of the cellular and molecular mechanisms underlying aging expands, so does the potential to intervene, repair, and rejuvenate. Yet, as with any frontier of scientific inquiry, age-reversal therapies come with their own set of promises and pitfalls.

The Lure of Age-Reversal

Imagine a world where the frailties of old age are mitigated, where age-related diseases such as Alzheimer's, cardiovascular disease, and osteoporosis are not just treated but reversed. This is the vision that drives age-reversal research. Several potential benefits of such therapies include:

- **Extended Healthspan:** The primary aim is not just to add years to life but to add life to years. Age-reversal could result in extended periods of vitality, activity, and health.

- **Reduced Burden of Age-Related Diseases:** From economic, emotional, and societal perspectives, age-related diseases place enormous burdens on individuals and healthcare systems. Reversing or delaying these diseases could lead to profound societal benefits.

- **Increased Lifespan:** While the primary goal is healthspan extension, successful age-reversal therapies might also lead to an increase in lifespan.

The Potential of Age-Reversal Therapies

Recent advancements provide tantalizing glimpses into the potential of age-reversal interventions:

- **Senolytics:** These are drugs that target senescent cells—cells that have lost their ability to function or divide but remain metabolically active and often produce inflammatory compounds. By removing these cells, researchers have noted improved health outcomes in animal models.

- **Stem Cell Therapies:** As we age, our reservoirs of stem cells—cells capable of turning into various cell types—deplete. Reintroducing stem cells could aid in tissue repair and regeneration.

- **Epigenetic Modulation:** As previously discussed, interventions targeting the epigenome, especially using molecules that can reset epigenetic markers, hold promise for age-reversal.

- **Metabolic Interventions:** Targeting fundamental metabolic pathways, such as mTOR and AMPK, with drugs like rapamycin and metformin, has shown potential in extending healthspan and, in some cases, lifespan in animals.

Challenges in Age-Reversal Therapies

Despite the potential, significant challenges need addressing:

- **Safety Concerns:** Any intervention at the cellular or molecular level carries inherent risks. There are concerns about potential side effects, especially over the long term. For instance, while senolytic drugs kill senescent cells, they might also harm healthy cells.

- **Complexity of Aging:** Aging is not driven by a single factor. It's a multifaceted process, influenced by genetics, environment, and stochastic events. Targeting one pathway might not yield comprehensive benefits.

- **Ethical and Societal Implications:** Longer lives and healthspans raise ethical questions. How would society adapt to longer-lived individuals? What are the implications for retirement, work, or intergenerational dynamics?

- **Accessibility:** There's a genuine concern that age-reversal therapies might become luxury goods, accessible only to the wealthy and deepening societal divides.

- **Unintended Consequences:** Nature maintains a balance, and interfering with fundamental processes like aging could have unforeseen repercussions. For instance, certain protective mechanisms that get activated with age might be suppressed, leading to unintended health issues.

The Way Forward

The challenges, though significant, are not insurmountable. To harness the full potential of age-reversal therapies, a multi-pronged approach is needed:

- **Holistic Research:** A focus on understanding the aging process in its entirety, rather than piecemeal, will yield more comprehensive insights.
- **Safety Trials:** Rigorous testing for safety, especially in the long term, is paramount.
- **Ethical Discourse:** Engaging ethicists, sociologists, and the general public in conversations about the implications of age-reversal is crucial.
- **Regulatory Frameworks:** Regulatory bodies need to evolve frameworks that facilitate the development and testing of age-reversal therapies while ensuring public safety.

Conclusion: The Horizon of Age-Reversal

The quest for age-reversal, a timeless human aspiration, stands on the cusp of scientific plausibility. As researchers unlock the secrets of our cells, the dream of reversing the clock inches closer to reality. While challenges lie ahead, the potential benefits for humanity — in terms of health, vitality, and longevity — make this one of the most exciting and consequential frontiers of modern science.

Ethical Considerations

As we march forward into the realm of potential age-reversal and lifespan extension, the ethical landscape becomes as intricate as the biological one. The possibility of modifying epigenetic markers to rejuvenate cells, delay aging, and extend life brings forth a series of profound ethical considerations that society, at large, must grapple with.

The Inequity of Access

The Cost of Innovation: The initial stages of any medical breakthrough tend to be expensive. If age-reversal therapies come to fruition, they might be out of reach for a significant portion of the population, especially in the early stages. This raises concerns about exacerbating existing health inequities.

The Socioeconomic Divide: The potential division between those who can afford these treatments and those who can't may lead to a societal divide, with a privileged subset of the population enjoying extended health and vitality while others face the natural ravages of time.

The Implications for Population and Resources

Overpopulation Concerns: If a significant portion of the global population has access to age-reversal therapies, we might see a spike in global population numbers. This could strain already limited resources like water, food, and energy.

Environmental Impact: The footprint of an ever-growing human population could exacerbate environmental challenges, including climate change, habitat destruction, and species extinction.

The Challenge of Longevity

Life's Natural Arc: While the promise of longer life is enticing, it prompts us to ask deep philosophical questions about the nature and quality of life. Does a longer life equate to a meaningful one? What are the psychological implications of living significantly longer than previous generations?

Interpersonal Dynamics: Longer lives could also impact family structures and relationships. How would human dynamics change if, for instance, five living generations coexisted instead of the typical three?

Redistribution of Life's Milestones

Career Implications: With an extended healthspan, would people retire at the same age? How would this impact job opportunities for younger generations? Would we experience career burnouts more frequently?

Education and Skill Acquisition: Lifelong learning might become the norm, with people going back to school multiple times during their extended lives.

The Nature of Medical Treatment

Prevention vs. Treatment: If we can treat age, one of the largest risk factors for many diseases, what becomes the primary role of healthcare? Would our medical paradigm shift more heavily towards prevention rather than treatment?

Allocation of Medical Resources: If significant resources are poured into age-reversal, would this divert necessary resources from other essential medical areas, especially those affecting the younger population?

Consent and Autonomy

Informed Decisions: Age-reversal therapies, especially in their infancy, would come with unknown long-term risks. How can patients give informed consent if even experts can't predict the long-term implications of these therapies?

The Role of Guardians: If these therapies show potential benefits for cognition and could potentially reverse cognitive decline, what are the ethical parameters around administering them to patients with dementia or similar conditions who can't provide consent?

The Morality of Playing with Time

Interfering with Nature: At a fundamental level, there's an ethical debate around whether humans should interfere with the natural aging process. Is it our place to play with the very fabric of existence?

Religious and Cultural Sensitivities: Various cultures and religions have beliefs centered around the sanctity of life, its natural progression, and the concept of an afterlife. Age-reversal therapies could challenge or contradict these deeply held beliefs.

Conclusion: Navigating the Ethical Maze

The science of epigenetic therapies and age-reversal is undoubtedly exciting, promising a future that once resided only in the realm of fantastical tales. However, with such promise comes responsibility. As we decode our epigenetic landscapes and unlock the secrets of time held within our cells, we must also engage in serious, collective ethical reflection. Science can answer the "how," but it's up to society to grapple with the "should." The interplay between these two questions will shape the trajectory of age-reversal therapies in the decades to come.

Chapter 9: Epigenetic Drugs and Longevity

Introduction to Drugs Targeting the Epigenome

The burgeoning field of epigenetics has ushered in a new era of medicine, emphasizing not just our genetic code, but the factors that dictate its expression. As our understanding of the epigenome deepens, so does our realization that it holds therapeutic promise, especially in the realm of longevity and age-associated diseases. Among the most promising avenues are drugs that target the epigenome. Before we delve into specific compounds and their potential implications, let's understand the fundamentals of epigenetic drugs and why they represent a paradigm shift in the way we approach medicine.

The Logic of Epigenetic Drugs

Beyond Genetic Mutations: Traditional drug discovery often focuses on genetic mutations as the root cause of many diseases. However, it's becoming clear that abnormal epigenetic modifications can be just as detrimental. Epigenetic drugs aim to correct these aberrant marks, restoring the regular functioning of genes without altering the DNA sequence itself.

Targeting the Root, Not Just the Symptom: Many of the age-related conditions, including cancers, arise due to epigenetic drift or dysregulation. By targeting these epigenetic changes, we address the disease at its source, rather than merely treating its symptoms.

Classes of Epigenetic Drugs

Histone Modifiers: Some of the first epigenetic drugs were developed to target histones, the proteins around which DNA is wound. By modulating the acetylation or methylation status of histones, these drugs can influence gene expression. HDAC inhibitors, for instance, are a class of drugs that prevent the removal of acetyl groups from histones, promoting a more open chromatin structure and altering gene expression.

DNA Methylation Modifiers: Another class of epigenetic drugs focuses on DNA methylation. By targeting the enzymes responsible for adding or removing methyl groups from DNA, these drugs can reactivate silenced genes or silence overly active ones.

Non-coding RNA Modulators: A more recent frontier in epigenetic drug discovery is the modulation of non-coding RNAs, which play critical roles in regulating gene expression and other cellular processes.

The Success Story: Epigenetic Drugs in Oncology

While the application of epigenetic drugs for longevity is still in its infancy, their potential has been vividly demonstrated in oncology. Cancers frequently arise from a combination of genetic mutations and epigenetic dysregulation. By targeting the latter, epigenetic drugs have achieved notable successes in treating specific types of cancers, setting the stage for broader applications in other age-associated diseases.

5-Azacytidine and 5-Aza-2'-deoxycytidine: These are DNA methyltransferase inhibitors, originally developed as cytotoxic agents but later found to have profound demethylating properties. They've been approved for the treatment of myelodysplastic syndromes, a group of bone marrow disorders.

HDAC Inhibitors: Several HDAC inhibitors, such as vorinostat and romidepsin, have received FDA approval for the treatment of cutaneous T cell lymphoma. Their success has spurred interest in investigating these compounds in other contexts.

Broad Spectrum vs. Specific Targeting

One of the challenges in developing epigenetic drugs is the decision between broad-spectrum drugs, which influence a wide array of epigenetic marks, and those that target a specific modification. While broad-spectrum drugs might be effective in conditions where multiple epigenetic aberrations exist, they also come with the risk of unintended side effects due to their wide-ranging impact. On the other hand, drugs with precise targets might offer fewer side effects but require a more in-depth understanding of the disease's epigenetic underpinnings.

Looking Ahead: The Potential for Longevity

While much of the current application of epigenetic drugs is in the realm of oncology, their potential application for longevity is tantalizing. As we've seen in earlier chapters, aging is accompanied by characteristic epigenetic shifts, some of which may drive the aging process itself. By modulating these changes, we may not only treat age-associated diseases but also potentially slow, halt, or even reverse aspects of the aging process.

In the subsequent sections, we'll delve deeper into specific drugs, their mechanisms of action, and the preclinical and clinical evidence supporting their role in promoting healthspan and lifespan. As with all medical interventions, it's essential to approach with both excitement and caution, balancing the promise of extended health with the imperative of ensuring safety and understanding long-term implications.

Current Applications in Cancer and Other Diseases

The epigenetic landscape of cells plays a pivotal role in determining gene expression profiles. When this landscape is altered, it can lead to a plethora of diseases, most notably cancer. Recognizing the profound impact of epigenetic changes on disease initiation and progression, researchers have been investigating drugs that can modify the epigenome as potential therapeutic interventions.

Here, we'll explore the current applications of these epigenetic drugs, with an emphasis on cancer and a few other notable diseases.

Epigenetic Drugs in Oncology

Cancer is fundamentally a disease of the genome. However, it's not just genetic mutations but also epigenetic alterations that drive cancer progression. Epigenetic drugs in oncology mainly fall into two categories: those targeting DNA methylation and those influencing histone modifications.

DNA Methylation Modifiers in Cancer:

- **5-Azacytidine (Vidaza) and Decitabine (Dacogen):** These are among the first FDA-approved epigenetic drugs. They're DNA methyltransferase inhibitors, reactivating genes that were silenced due to hypermethylation. Both have shown efficacy in treating myelodysplastic syndromes.

Histone Modification Modifiers in Cancer:

- **HDAC Inhibitors:** Several HDAC inhibitors, like vorinostat (Zolinza) and romidepsin (Istodax), have been approved for cutaneous T cell lymphoma. By altering histone acetylation patterns, these drugs influence the chromatin structure and, subsequently, gene expression.
- **BET Inhibitors:** This is a newer class targeting the bromodomain and extraterminal (BET) proteins, which recognize acetylated histones. They show promise in several cancers, including leukemia and solid tumors, by disrupting the expression of critical oncogenes.

Epigenetic Drugs in Neurological Diseases

Recent research suggests that epigenetic mechanisms play roles in various neurological diseases, from neurodegenerative conditions like Alzheimer's to psychiatric disorders like depression.

- **HDAC Inhibitors in Huntington's Disease:** Preclinical studies have indicated that HDAC inhibitors can increase the acetylation of histones linked to the Huntington's gene, potentially reducing the production of the toxic protein fragment that causes the disease.
- **DNA Methylation Modifiers in Rett Syndrome:** Rett syndrome, a severe neurological disorder, has been associated with MECP2 gene mutations. Drugs that modulate DNA methylation have shown promise in animal models, potentially paving the way for human applications.

Epigenetic Drugs in Autoimmune Diseases

Autoimmune diseases, where the body's immune system attacks its own cells, have also been associated with epigenetic alterations.

- **Rheumatoid Arthritis:** DNA methylation patterns in cells from patients with rheumatoid arthritis differ significantly from healthy controls. Epigenetic drugs that modify these patterns could potentially offer therapeutic benefits.
- **Lupus:** HDAC inhibitors have shown promise in animal models of lupus, hinting at their potential applications in human patients.

Epigenetic Drugs in Cardiovascular Diseases

Cardiovascular diseases remain the leading cause of death worldwide. Emerging evidence suggests that epigenetic mechanisms play a role in conditions like atherosclerosis, heart failure, and hypertension.

- **HDAC Inhibitors in Heart Failure:** Preclinical studies have shown that specific HDAC inhibitors can prevent pathological cardiac remodeling, a major factor in heart failure.

Challenges and Considerations

While the promise of epigenetic drugs is immense, several challenges persist:

1. **Specificity:** Most epigenetic drugs are broad-spectrum, influencing a wide array of targets. This can lead to unintended side effects.

2. **Durability:** Unlike genetic mutations, epigenetic marks are dynamic. It remains to be seen how long the effects of epigenetic drugs last and whether repeated dosing might be required.

3. **Combination Therapies:** Given the complex nature of diseases like cancer, combining epigenetic drugs with other treatments might offer the best therapeutic outcomes.

Concluding Thoughts

Epigenetic drugs represent a new frontier in medicine. Their ability to modulate gene expression without altering the underlying DNA sequence offers a novel approach to treating diseases that have remained elusive to traditional therapeutics. While most current applications are in oncology, it's evident that the potential of these drugs spans across various medical disciplines. As research advances, we can anticipate a growing list of diseases that might benefit from these groundbreaking drugs.

The Potential for Lifespan Extension through Pharmacology

The quest for the proverbial "fountain of youth" has captivated humanity for centuries. While the idea of an elixir that grants eternal youth remains a myth, modern science has made significant strides in understanding the molecular and cellular determinants of aging. One of the most promising areas of research is pharmacology and its potential role in extending lifespan. This section delves into the current understanding of pharmacological interventions that might impact aging and longevity.

Molecular Targets of Aging

Aging is a multifaceted process, influenced by genetics, environment, lifestyle, and stochastic factors. At the molecular level, several pathways have been identified as being intimately linked to the aging process:

- **mTOR (Mechanistic Target of Rapamycin) Pathway:** Integral for cell growth and metabolism, the mTOR pathway has emerged as a critical determinant of lifespan in various organisms, from yeast to mammals.
- **Sirtuins:** A family of proteins that regulate cellular health, sirtuins can increase lifespan in many organisms when activated.
- **AMP-activated protein kinase (AMPK):** Acts as an energy sensor and regulator, maintaining cellular energy homeostasis. Activation can mimic caloric restriction benefits, which has been shown to extend lifespan.

Pharmacological Interventions Targeting Aging Pathways

Several compounds have shown promise in targeting these pathways, potentially extending lifespan:

- **Rapamycin:** An inhibitor of the mTOR pathway, rapamycin has extended lifespan in a myriad of organisms. In mice, rapamycin treatment has led to a significant increase in lifespan, even when administered late in life. The drug is already FDA-approved for other indications, making it a prime candidate for human aging studies.
- **NAD+ Boosters:** NAD+ is a coenzyme crucial for many cellular processes, and its levels decline with age. Compounds like NMN (nicotinamide mononucleotide) and NR (nicotinamide riboside) can boost NAD+ levels, activating sirtuins and potentially extending lifespan.
- **Metformin:** A widely-used diabetic drug, metformin activates AMPK and has been associated with increased lifespan in animal models. Observational studies in humans suggest that diabetic patients on metformin tend to live longer than

non-diabetics not on the drug, sparking interest in its anti-aging potential.

- **Resveratrol:** Found in red wine, resveratrol activates sirtuins. While its effects on lifespan in mammals are still debated, it has shown potential in improving healthspan, the period of life spent in good health.

Translating Findings to Human Longevity

While these compounds show promise, translating findings from model organisms to humans poses challenges:

1. **Dosage and Safety:** Determining the correct dosage that elicits anti-aging effects without causing adverse reactions is challenging. For instance, the amount of resveratrol given to mice to observe benefits far exceeds what a human can consume from wine or supplements.

2. **Biomarkers of Aging:** Aging isn't a disease, making it challenging to identify precise endpoints for clinical trials. Researchers need reliable biomarkers to assess the efficacy of anti-aging drugs.

3. **Long-term Effects:** Interventions might have benefits in the short term but detrimental effects in the long run. Comprehensive long-term studies are necessary before declaring any drug as a true "anti-aging" compound.

Ethical Considerations

Pharmacological interventions for lifespan extension aren't without ethical dilemmas:

- **Resource Implications:** If individuals live significantly longer, it could strain resources, especially if the extended life isn't accompanied by improved healthspan.
- **Access and Equity:** There's the potential for anti-aging treatments to be accessible only to the wealthy, exacerbating societal inequities.

- **Nature of Human Existence:** Philosophical debates arise about the very nature of life and whether humans should interfere with the natural aging process.

Concluding Thoughts

The potential of pharmacology in lifespan extension is an exciting frontier in biogerontology. While the path is fraught with challenges, both scientific and ethical, the rewards are immense. The aim is not just to add years to life but, more importantly, life to years. If pharmacology can help achieve a longer healthspan, where individuals live longer with vitality and free from chronic diseases, it could revolutionize the very way we perceive and experience aging.

Chapter 10: Challenges and Frontiers in Epigenetic Longevity Research

The Complexity of the Epigenome and its Implications

Epigenetics, derived from the Greek word "epi-" meaning "over" or "above", has introduced a new dimension to our understanding of genetics. While genetics involves the study of genes and their sequences, epigenetics delves into the factors that influence gene activity without changing the DNA sequence. The epigenome, composed of all the epigenetic marks across our genome, offers an intricate layer of regulation. Its complexity and dynamism pose both challenges and opportunities for the field of longevity research.

Epigenome: A Dynamic Landscape

Unlike the relatively static genome, the epigenome is in constant flux. It can be influenced by:

- **Environmental Factors:** Factors like diet, stress, and exposure to toxins can alter epigenetic marks.
- **Developmental Stages:** As organisms grow and differentiate, their epigenetic marks change to accommodate new cellular roles.
- **Disease States:** Many diseases, especially cancers, are associated with epigenetic changes.

This dynamism means that our epigenetic profile at birth is significantly different from that in adulthood or old age. The fluidity of

the epigenome makes studying it more challenging but also introduces the possibility of reversing or modifying undesirable marks.

Implications for Disease and Aging

The epigenome's complexity means that even small changes can
ripple across the genome with broad effects. For example:

- **Silencing of Tumor Suppressor Genes:** In cancer, certain
  epigenetic changes can silence genes that typically prevent
  uncontrolled growth.
- **Activation of Normally Silent Genes:** Some genes meant to
  be off might become activated due to epigenetic alterations,
  leading to diseases.
- **Influence on Aging:** As organisms age, the epigenome accumulates changes that can influence healthspan and lifespan.

Given these profound effects, understanding the epigenome
could lead to breakthroughs in treatments for diseases and potentially anti-aging interventions.

Challenges in Deciphering the Epigenome

Studying the epigenome is not without its challenges:

- **Interindividual Variation:** Even identical twins, with the same
  genetic makeup, can have different epigenomes. This variability makes it challenging to identify consistent epigenetic
  patterns.
- **Cell-type Specificity:** The epigenome varies across different
  cell types. A liver cell's epigenetic marks differ from that of
  a brain cell. Thus, comprehensive epigenetic studies require
  analysis of specific cell types, complicating large-scale research.
- **Cause vs. Consequence:** Determining whether epigenetic
  changes are the cause of a disease/aging or a result is challenging. This differentiation is crucial for therapeutic interventions.

Opportunities in Epigenetic Interventions

The dynamic nature of the epigenome offers hope for interventions:

- **Reversibility:** Unlike genetic mutations, epigenetic changes are potentially reversible. Drugs that can modify epigenetic marks might restore normal gene function.
- **Early Detection:** Epigenetic changes can precede visible disease symptoms. Identifying these early markers could lead to preventative treatments.
- **Personalized Medicine:** Given the individual-specific nature of the epigenome, treatments can be tailored to an individual's epigenetic profile, maximizing efficacy.

Looking Forward: Future of Epigenetic Longevity Research

The intricate dance of epigenetic marks on our DNA holds secrets yet to be unraveled. Key areas to watch for in future research include:

- **Epigenetic Clocks:** The discovery that certain DNA methylation patterns correlate with age has led to the concept of an "epigenetic clock." Understanding this clock's mechanics might offer insights into aging processes and how to potentially reverse them.
- **Epigenetic Therapies:** While still in their infancy, drugs targeting the epigenome are emerging. Their potential in treating diseases and promoting longevity remains an exciting frontier.
- **Interplay with Genetics:** How the genome and epigenome interact, influencing each other in the context of disease and aging, will be a vital area of study.

In conclusion, the epigenome's complexity presents both challenges and opportunities for longevity research. As technology advances and our understanding deepens, the potential to harness the epigenome's dynamism for health and longevity becomes increasingly tangible. The next decade promises exciting revelations and innovations in this space, bringing science closer to unlocking the mysteries of aging and, possibly, the keys to longer, healthier lives.

Differentiating Between Causation and Correlation in Research

In the realm of scientific research, particularly in the study of epigenetics and longevity, a crucial challenge is distinguishing between causation and correlation. This differentiation is paramount because it determines the inference we make from data and how we apply that knowledge. Misinterpreting correlation for causation can lead to ineffective treatments or misguided health recommendations. As such, understanding this distinction is pivotal for both researchers and those consuming scientific findings.

What is Correlation?

Correlation refers to a relationship or association between two or more variables. When one variable changes, there's a predictable change in the other variable. It's quantified by the correlation coefficient, which ranges from -1 to 1. A value closer to 1 implies a strong positive correlation, meaning as one variable increases, the other also does. A value closer to -1 implies a strong negative correlation: as one variable increases, the other decreases. A value near 0 suggests little to no relationship.

Example in Epigenetics: If studies find that individuals with a specific epigenetic mark also tend to have a longer lifespan, there's a correlation between that mark and longevity.

What is Causation?

Causation implies that a change in one variable is responsible for a change in another. It goes beyond mere association to signify a direct effect. If A causes B, then altering A will result in a predictable change in B.

Example in Epigenetics: If removing or introducing a particular epigenetic mark in a controlled setting directly leads to a change in lifespan, then that mark causally influences longevity.

Challenges in Distinguishing Correlation from Causation

Several factors make it challenging to differentiate between the two:

- **Confounding Variables:** These are external factors that might influence the observed relationship. For example, if a specific epigenetic mark correlates with longevity but is also associated with a healthy diet, it might be the diet, not the mark, causing increased lifespan.

- **Bidirectional Causation:** Sometimes A affects B, but B also affects A. Determining the primary causal factor becomes tricky in such scenarios.

- **Coincidental Correlation:** Two variables might correlate purely by chance, without any underlying causal relationship.

Why it Matters in Epigenetic Longevity Research

Directing Interventions: Misinterpreting correlation for causation can lead to misguided interventions. If we incorrectly believe an epigenetic mark causes longevity, resources might be wasted targeting it, only to find it has no effect.

Understanding Mechanisms: Grasping the underlying causes of longevity can lead to breakthrough treatments and preventive measures. If we only understand correlations, we might miss vital insights into the biology of aging.

Patient Expectations: People hoping for anti-aging treatments rely on accurate interpretations of research. Mistaking correlation for causation can lead to false hope or misinformed decisions.

Strategies to Determine Causation

Researchers employ several methods to infer causation:

- **Randomized Controlled Trials (RCTs):** Participants are randomly assigned to different groups. One receives the intervention, while the other(s) do not, helping to eliminate confounding variables. If a significant difference emerges, it provides strong evidence of causation.

- **Longitudinal Studies:** These track participants over time, observing how changes in one variable (like an epigenetic mark) might lead to changes in another (like health outcomes).

- **Mechanistic Studies:** These delve deep into biological processes, often at the cellular or molecular level, to understand how one factor might directly influence another.

Caveats and Considerations

Even with rigorous research methods, it's essential to remain cautious:

- **Complex Interplay:** Especially in epigenetics, myriad factors interact in intricate ways. One epigenetic mark might influence another, which in turn affects gene expression, which then impacts cell function, and so on.

- **External Validity:** Just because a causal relationship is found in a specific setting (e.g., a lab or among a particular population) doesn't mean it will generalize everywhere.

- **Evolution of Knowledge:** Science is a dynamic field. What's believed to be causative today might be understood as merely correlative tomorrow as new information emerges.

In conclusion, while correlational insights offer valuable starting points, digging deeper to understand causation is crucial for tangible progress in epigenetic longevity research. As we embark on the frontier of understanding how epigenetic marks influence aging, grounding our conclusions in robust, causative evidence is not just an academic exercise; it's a commitment to effective, evidence-based interventions that can genuinely enhance human health and lifespan.

The Future Trajectory of Epigenetics and Longevity Studies

The intersection of epigenetics and longevity has witnessed a meteoric rise in research interest. The potential to decode the complex relationship between our epigenome and aging promises not just a deeper understanding of biology but also revolutionary interventions in health and medicine. As we reflect upon the trajectory of this discipline, it's crucial to envision what lies ahead. Here, we explore the prospective directions, breakthroughs, and challenges that might shape the future of epigenetics and longevity studies.

Expanding the Scope of Research

The foundation laid by current studies will likely catalyze a more expansive exploration into:

- **Diverse Populations:** Much of the early research has focused on specific populations. The future holds a broader study encompassing varied ethnicities, geographies, and lifestyles to understand the universal and unique epigenetic factors affecting aging.

- **Integration with Other Disciplines:** Epigenetics doesn't operate in isolation. Collaborations with fields like metabolomics, proteomics, and computational biology will enhance the depth and breadth of findings.

- **Environmental Interactions:** We've just scratched the surface of understanding how external factors like pollution, radiation, and even social interactions impact our epigenome and, in turn, aging.

Technological Advancements

Technology has always been a driving force in scientific exploration. In epigenetics and longevity:

- **High-Throughput Sequencing:** The capacity to sequence DNA faster and more affordably will allow for large-scale projects, potentially mapping the entire epigenome across various life stages and conditions.

- **AI and Machine Learning:** Handling the vast data sets in epigenetics requires computational power and algorithms capable of discerning patterns and predicting outcomes.
- **Advanced Imaging Techniques:** Observing epigenetic changes in real-time, especially in living organisms, will be pivotal in understanding the dynamic nature of the epigenome.

Breakthroughs in Interventions

As our knowledge deepens, the potential for tangible applications grows:

- **Epigenetic Therapies:** Targeting specific epigenetic marks to delay aging or reverse age-related diseases could become standard practice. This is not just about extending life but enhancing its quality.
- **Personalized Medicine:** Recognizing that each individual's epigenome is unique, treatments and preventive measures tailored to personal epigenetic profiles might become the norm.
- **Diet and Lifestyle Recommendations:** With deeper insights into how daily choices influence the epigenome and aging, evidence-based guidelines can help people make informed decisions for healthier, longer lives.

Ethical and Societal Implications

The profound impacts of epigenetics on longevity aren't just biological but touch upon ethical and societal facets:

- **Access to Treatments:** With potential life-extending therapies on the horizon, who gets access and at what cost becomes a significant concern.
- **Societal Structures:** If significantly extending human life becomes a reality, it will reshape societal structures, from employment and retirement to relationships and population dynamics.

- **Genetic Privacy:** As more becomes known about an individual's epigenome and its implications for health and longevity, issues around data privacy, insurance, and employment decisions emerge.

Potential Challenges

The path forward isn't without obstacles:

- **Complexity of the Epigenome:** The sheer intricacy of epigenetic interactions means that there's no simple formula for understanding or manipulating it.

- **Safety and Unintended Consequences:** Any intervention, especially at the epigenetic level, holds the risk of unforeseen side effects, which might manifest immediately or decades later.

- **Distinguishing Hype from Reality:** With the surge in interest around anti-aging, there's potential for overhyped claims, misinterpretations, and commercial pressures that could skew research priorities.

Collaboration and Open Science

The scale and significance of exploring the epigenetic determinants of aging demand a collaborative approach:

- **Global Collaborations:** Epigenetic changes aren't confined by borders. Cross-country partnerships can provide diverse datasets and a holistic understanding.

- **Public and Private Partnerships:** Combining the resources of governments, academia, and industry can accelerate research and application.

- **Open Science:** Making research findings, datasets, and methodologies freely accessible can spur innovation, validate findings, and ensure that progress benefits humanity at large.

In conclusion, the journey of understanding the interplay between epigenetics and longevity is filled with promise and challenges. As we chart the trajectory of this field, it's clear that the future isn't just about adding years to life but adding life to years.

The implications are profound, reshaping our understanding of biology, redefining the potentials of medicine, and challenging our societal constructs. As with any frontier, the path is uncertain and complex, but the potential rewards – healthier, more vibrant lives for all – make it a journey worth undertaking.

Conclusion

Summarizing Key Insights from the Book

As we stand at the crossroads of knowledge and discovery, this book has embarked on an explorative journey into the intricate world of epigenetics and its undeniable link to human longevity. As we wrap up this literary journey, let's distill the core insights and revelations we've garnered along the way.

The Multifaceted Epigenome

Key Insight: Beyond our genes, the epigenome provides an additional layer of instruction, dictating how, when, and where genes should function. It's not just about the 'what' (DNA) but also the 'how' (epigenetics).

- **The Epigenetic Landscape:** Our understanding of genetics has been dramatically enriched by the discovery of DNA methylation, histone modifications, and non-coding RNA, elements that determine the unique expression of our genes.
- **Dynamic Nature:** Far from being static, the epigenome is a fluid and adaptive interface, reacting to internal and external stimuli and evolving with age.

A Biological Clock Within

Key Insight: The epigenome might hold the key to understanding our biological age, a more profound indicator of health than chronological age.

- **DNA Methylation & Age:** By assessing patterns of DNA methylation, scientists have developed epigenetic clocks, potentially predicting disease risk and even lifespan.
- **Health Implications:** This biological clock doesn't merely tell time; it might signal health disparities, disease predispositions, and more.

Lifestyle's Mark on the Epigenome

Key Insight: Our daily choices, from the foods we consume to our physical activities, have a tangible impact on our epigenetic profile, influencing how our genes are expressed.

- **Diet & DNA Methylation:** Diets can either hasten or delay epigenetic aging, emphasizing the importance of nutritional choices.
- **Physical Activity's Rejuvenating Touch:** Exercise, in its many forms, can potentially reverse epigenetic aging, offering a protective shield against age-associated diseases.
- **Smoking, Alcohol, and Stress:** These lifestyle factors leave a detectable footprint on the epigenome, influencing not only our health but also the health of subsequent generations.

Starvation's Silver Lining

Key Insight: Caloric restriction, paradoxically, might be a key to extended healthspan, with epigenetics playing a central role.

- **Across Species:** From yeast to primates, caloric restriction appears to extend lifespan, hinting at a universal biological mechanism.
- **Linking Diet & Longevity:** The molecular pathways activated by reduced calorie intake intersect with epigenetic mechanisms, offering a fresh perspective on aging.

The Histone-Gene Tango

Key Insight: Histones, proteins around which DNA winds, play an instrumental role in gene regulation, and their modifications offer clues about aging and longevity.

- **Expression through Alteration:** Histone modifications can activate or suppress genes, influencing processes from cell growth to apoptosis.
- **Histones & Aging:** Age-related changes in histone modifications might be both a result of and a contributor to cellular aging.

Heredity Beyond Genes

Key Insight: Epigenetic information can be passed down generations, challenging traditional notions of inheritance and evolution.

- **Transgenerational Epigenetics:** Phenomena like famine's lingering effects highlight the potential for environmental factors to impact descendants epigenetically.
- **Family Health Ties:** Understanding this can offer insights into familial disease patterns and predispositions.

Decoding Disease through Epigenetics

Key Insight: Many age-related diseases, from Alzheimer's to cardiovascular ailments, display epigenetic alterations, offering new therapeutic avenues.

- **Epigenetic Disease Markers:** Epigenetic changes might be early indicators, predictors, or even drivers of diseases.
- **Therapeutic Potential:** Epigenetic interventions could revolutionize treatment, management, and prevention of diseases.

Future Horizons in Epigenetic Therapies

Key Insight: We stand at the cusp of potential breakthroughs in reversing aging and disease progression through epigenetic therapies.

- **Rejuvenation Research:** Preliminary studies hint at the possibility of not just slowing but reversing aging markers.
- **Ethical Conundrums:** The power to modify epigenetic patterns brings with it ethical challenges concerning consent, equity, and unforeseen consequences.

Drugs Targeting the Epigenome

Key Insight: Pharmacology is tapping into the epigenome's potential, with drugs that can modify epigenetic patterns, offering hope for numerous conditions, including aging.

- **Cancer & Beyond**: While cancer therapy is the current primary application, the horizon looks promising for a broader range of diseases, possibly even aging itself.

The Research Road Ahead

Key Insight: The journey of discovery in epigenetics and longevity is paved with promise, complexities, and ethical quandaries.

- **Interpreting Findings**: Discerning causation from correlation is vital, ensuring we act on concrete science rather than coincidences.
- **Future's Beacon**: With technology, collaboration, and ethics guiding the way, the future of epigenetics and longevity research beams with potential.

In this intricate dance of genes, environment, choices, and time, epigenetics offers a fresh lens through which we can understand and influence the process of aging. As we peer into the future, armed with the insights from this book, the possibilities are not just scientifically exhilarating but also deeply human. The quest isn't merely for extended life but enriched life, where every moment counts.

The Holistic Approach to Understanding and Influencing Human Aging through Epigenetics

The profound quest to understand the underpinnings of human aging and to influence its trajectory has been a cornerstone of scientific exploration. In recent years, the focus has pivoted from a purely genetic paradigm to the more nuanced and dynamic realm of epigenetics. The epigenetic lens not only uncovers new dimensions of understanding aging but also emphasizes a holistic approach that encapsulates our genes, environment, lifestyle, and choices.

The Intersection of Genes, Environment, and Lifestyle

Key Insight: The dance between our genetic code and the influences from our environment and lifestyle choices form the essence of the epigenetic paradigm.

- **Nature and Nurture in Cohesion**: While our genetic blueprint provides a foundational structure, epigenetic modifications elucidate how environmental factors and personal choices can shift the expression of these genes.
- **Adaptability and Flexibility**: The dynamic nature of epigenetic modifications highlights the body's ability to adapt and respond to varying conditions, offering insights into potential interventions.

An Integrated Approach to Aging

Key Insight: Aging is not a singular, linear process but an amalgamation of genetic predispositions, environmental exposures, and cumulative lifestyle decisions.

- **The Multifaceted Aging Process**: The accumulation of epigenetic changes over time forms a complex tapestry of modifications that might contribute to aging and age-related diseases. These changes can be influenced by myriad factors, from diet and exercise to stress and exposure to toxins.
- **Feedback Loops**: The interconnectedness of these factors creates feedback loops. For instance, a healthful diet might promote favorable epigenetic changes, which in turn might enhance overall well-being, creating a positive feedback loop.

Embracing Complexity and Interconnectedness

Key Insight: To truly grasp and influence aging, we need to adopt a systems biology approach, viewing the body as an interconnected whole rather than isolated components.

- **Beyond Silos**: Traditional research often studies biological processes in isolation. In contrast, epigenetics underscores the importance of studying interactions between genes, cells, organs, and systems within the broader context of external influences.

- **The Ripple Effect**: An intervention in one aspect of our lives or health might have cascading effects throughout the system. Understanding these ripples can guide holistic interventions.

Proactive and Preventative Interventions

Key Insight: Epigenetics not only offers insights into the causes and progression of aging but also emphasizes proactive and preventive measures.

- **Anticipatory Health**: Recognizing the early epigenetic markers of disease or accelerated aging can guide interventions even before overt symptoms manifest. This proactive approach shifts the focus from disease treatment to disease prevention.
- **Personalized Medicine**: Epigenetic insights might pave the way for more personalized health strategies, tailored to an individual's unique epigenetic profile and environmental exposures.

Cultivating a Holistic Lifestyle

Key Insight: The lifestyle choices we make today have far-reaching implications on our epigenetic landscape, influencing our health trajectory and aging process.

- **Mindful Living**: Being aware of the foods we eat, our physical activity, our stress levels, and our overall lifestyle can be instrumental in shaping a healthful epigenetic profile.
- **Integrative Health**: Complementing modern medicine with traditional practices, mindfulness techniques, and holistic wellness strategies might offer a comprehensive approach to healthy aging.

Embracing the Bigger Picture

Key Insight: Epigenetics is a reminder that we are not mere passive recipients of our genetic inheritance but active participants in shaping our health destiny.

- **The Interplay of Factors:** The intertwined nature of genetics, environment, and lifestyle offers both challenges and opportunities. While there are factors beyond our control, the agency lies in leveraging what we can influence.
- **A Collaborative Future:** Bridging the gaps between various scientific disciplines, from genetics and biology to psychology and environmental science, can foster a multidisciplinary approach to aging research and interventions.

In essence, the epigenetic perspective on aging offers a holistic, integrated, and empowering framework. It reaffirms the age-old wisdom that life is an intricate balance of destiny and choice, of genes and environments, of individual actions and collective influences. By embracing this holistic approach, we stand at the precipice of not just understanding but also redefining the boundaries of human aging, aiming for a life that's not just longer, but also richer and more fulfilling.

Hope and Potential for Future Breakthroughs

As we venture deeper into the intricacies of epigenetics and human aging, we're ushered into an era replete with hope and anticipation. The revelations in epigenetics, and its intertwining with longevity, represent not just a scientific milestone but a beacon of optimism for what the future might hold. This conclusion encapsulates the burgeoning hope and the profound potential for pioneering breakthroughs in the coming decades.

From Understanding to Intervention

Key Insight: Our evolving understanding of epigenetics is gradually pivoting from mere observation to actionable interventions.

- **The Power of Knowledge**: The past few decades have seen an explosion in our comprehension of the epigenome. This foundational knowledge sets the stage for the next leap—using this understanding to devise interventions, both preventive and therapeutic.
- **Blueprint to Action**: The epigenetic mechanisms underlying aging and age-related diseases provide tangible targets for therapeutic approaches, opening the doors to novel drug developments and non-pharmacological strategies.

The Advent of Precision Medicine

Key Insight: Epigenetics brings us closer to the dream of precision medicine, where interventions are tailor-made to the individual's unique genetic and epigenetic profile.

- **Beyond One-size-fits-all**: The traditional approach to medicine often prescribes generalized treatments. With epigenetic insights, there's a burgeoning potential for treatments fine-tuned to individual needs and predispositions.
- **Personalized Longevity Plans**: In the near future, it's conceivable that individuals could have bespoke longevity strategies, meticulously crafted based on their epigenetic clocks, lifestyle, and environmental exposures.

Rejuvenation and Age Reversal

Key Insight: One of the most tantalizing prospects of epigenetic research is the potential for age reversal, turning back the biological clock.

- **More than Science Fiction**: Preliminary research in animal models has shown that it's possible, at least to some extent, to reverse signs of aging through targeted epigenetic interventions.
- **Redefining Aging**: If these findings can be translated to humans, we might be on the brink of not just extending lifespan but enhancing the quality of life in our later years, mitigating or even reversing age-related declines.

Cross-disciplinary Synergies

Key Insight: The future of epigenetic longevity research lies in fostering collaborations across disciplines, integrating insights from genetics, biology, medicine, technology, and even socioeconomics.

- **Harmonizing Diverse Fields:** The complex nature of the epigenome and its influencers necessitates a collaborative approach, pooling expertise from diverse scientific landscapes.
- **Technological Enablers:** Advancements in AI, machine learning, and data analytics offer powerful tools to dissect the vast and intricate datasets of epigenetics, accelerating discoveries and applications.

An Ethical Compass for the Journey Ahead

Key Insight: As with any groundbreaking scientific domain, the journey into epigenetics and longevity must be navigated with an ethical compass.

- **Inclusive Progress:** The potential benefits of epigenetic interventions should be accessible to all, avoiding disparities where only a privileged few reap the rewards of scientific advancements.
- **Balancing Enthusiasm with Caution:** While the promise of epigenetic-based interventions is exhilarating, it's crucial to tread with caution, ensuring rigorous testing and evaluation to ascertain safety and efficacy.

A Hopeful Horizon

Key Insight: The horizon of epigenetic research is radiant with hope, hinting at a future where aging is better understood, more gracefully navigated, and perhaps, even malleably influenced.

- **A New Paradigm of Aging:** The narrative of inevitable decline associated with aging might shift towards one of empowerment, where individuals have the tools and knowledge to influence their aging trajectories.

- **A Lifespan Filled with Life:** The ultimate aspiration isn't just about adding years to life but infusing those added years with vibrancy, health, and fulfillment.

In closing, the confluence of epigenetics and longevity research stands as a testament to human curiosity, ingenuity, and the perennial quest for betterment. While challenges lie ahead, they're dwarfed by the immense potential and the luminous hope that lights the path. As we stand on this precipice, looking into the future, it's a future shimmering with promise, potential, and the dream of a better, longer, and healthier life for all.

Appendix A: Glossary of Terms

The following is a compilation of crucial terms and concepts that have been introduced throughout the book. This glossary serves as a quick reference for readers, helping to elucidate the complex language of epigenetics and longevity.

A

Acetylation: The process by which an acetyl group is covalently attached to a molecule, often a protein. In the context of histones, acetylation usually leads to a more relaxed chromatin structure, facilitating gene expression.

B

Base Pair (bp): Two chemical bases bonded to one another forming a rung of the DNA ladder. The DNA molecule consists of two strands, each strand consisting of a sequence of bases. These bases are adenine (A), cytosine (C), guanine (G), and thymine (T).

C

Chromatin: The material of which chromosomes are made. It consists of protein, RNA, and DNA.

CpG Island: Regions with a high frequency of CpG sites. In the context of DNA methylation, CpG islands in promoter regions are often associated with gene regulation.

D

DNA (Deoxyribonucleic Acid): The molecule carrying genetic instructions for the development, functioning, growth, and reproduction of all known organisms and many viruses.

DNA Methylation: The addition of a methyl group to the DNA molecule, often leading to the repression of gene transcription.

E

Epigenetics: The study of changes in organisms caused by modification of gene expression rather than alteration of the genetic code itself.

Epigenome: The complete description of all the chemical modifications to the DNA and histone proteins of an organism.

H

Histone: A protein that DNA wraps around in the chromosomes of eukaryotic cells. Modifications to histones can affect gene expression.

Histone Modification: Chemical changes to the histone protein that can affect gene expression. These include methylation, acetylation, phosphorylation, and others.

L

Long Non-coding RNA (lncRNA): A type of RNA molecule that does not encode a protein but can play critical roles in regulating gene expression.

M

Methyl Group: A chemical group derived from methane. In the context of DNA, the addition of a methyl group (methylation) often represses gene transcription.

P

Phenotype: The set of observable characteristics or traits of an organism. The phenotype results from the expression of an organism's genes as well as the influence of environmental factors and possible interactions between the two.

Promoter: A region of DNA that initiates transcription of a particular gene. Promoters are located near the transcription start sites of genes, upstream on the DNA.

R

RNA (Ribonucleic Acid): A molecule similar to DNA that plays vital roles in coding, decoding, regulation, and expression of genes.

S

Sirtuins: A family of proteins that play roles in aging, inflammation, transcription, cellular health, and more. They can be influenced by dietary habits like caloric restriction.

T

Transcription: The process by which a specific segment of DNA is copied into RNA by the enzyme RNA polymerase.

Transgenerational Epigenetic Inheritance: The transmission of information from one generation of an organism to the next (e.g., parent-child transmission) that affects the traits of offspring without alteration of the primary structure of DNA (i.e., the sequence of nucleotides)—in other words, epigenetically.

U

Ubiquitination: A process that involves adding a ubiquitin protein to a substrate protein. It can regulate the degradation, cellular localization, or activity of proteins.

This glossary offers readers a foundation, but it is by no means exhaustive. The field of epigenetics, intertwined with the vast landscape of biology, continuously evolves, bringing forth new terminologies and concepts. The dedicated reader is encouraged to delve deeper, exploring beyond this appendix to grasp the nuances and intricacies of this fascinating realm.

Appendix B: Resources for Further Reading

The journey through the intricate maze of epigenetics and its profound impact on human longevity doesn't end with this book. Those passionate about digging deeper into the subject matter are encouraged to explore a curated list of resources for further reading, spanning seminal works, academic reviews, and groundbreaking research articles. Each provides a unique lens through which to view and understand the expanding field of epigenetics.

Books

1. "The Epigenetics Revolution: How Modern Biology is Rewriting Our Understanding of Genetics, Disease, and Inheritance" by Nessa Carey

   - Carey's work provides a comprehensive look at the transformative role of epigenetics in modern biology. An excellent read for both novices and seasoned scientists.

2. "The Deepest Well: Healing the Long-Term Effects of Childhood Adversity" by Nadine Burke Harris

   - This book delves into the intersections of stress, childhood traumas, and epigenetic changes, emphasizing the profound impacts on long-term health and well-being.

3. "Epigenetic Markers" by David Allis and Thomas Jenuwein

   - An academic text offering a deep dive into various epigenetic markers and their roles in health and disease.

Research Journals and Articles

1. **Nature Reviews Genetics**

   - A prestigious journal offering reviews on the latest developments in the field of genetics, including epigenetics.

2. **"DNA methylation age of human tissues and cell types" by Steve Horvath**

   - A landmark paper detailing the development and validation of the epigenetic clock.

3. **"Histone modifications at human enhancers reflect global cell-type-specific gene expression" by Nathaniel D. Heintzman et al.**

   - This article provides insights into the role of histone modifications in regulating gene expression specific to cell types.

4. **"Transgenerational epigenetic inheritance: myths and mechanisms" by David M. Evans, Sarah E. Medland, and Naomi R. Wray**

   - A critical review of the mechanisms and evidence for transgenerational epigenetic inheritance.

Websites and Online Platforms

1. **Epigenetics Literacy Project (http://www.epiliteracy.com)**

   - A platform dedicated to educating the public about epigenetics. The site features articles, resources, and discussions about the latest in epigenetics research.

2. **DNA Methylation Database (http://www.dnamethdb.com)**

   - A curated database offering information on DNA methylation patterns across various species, tissues, and diseases.

3. The Roadmap Epigenomics Project

- An extensive project aimed at defining epigenomic changes in primary human tissues and cells. The website - http://www.roadmapepigenomics.org - offers tools, data sets, and publications.

Podcasts and Webinars

1. "Epigenetics: A New Frontier in Medicine"–Webinar by Dr. Andrew Feinberg

- A detailed webinar exploring the implications of epigenetics in the realm of medicine, touching on topics from cancer to neurological diseases.

2. The Epigenetics Podcast

- A series featuring discussions with leading researchers in the field of epigenetics, providing insights into the latest developments, methodologies, and discoveries.

Organizations and Institutes

1. The International Human Epigenome Consortium (IHEC)

- A global consortium with the mission to decode the human epigenome. IHEC supports research projects, events, and publications focused on understanding the epigenetic underpinnings of health and disease.

2. Epigenetics Society

- An organization that brings together researchers, educators, and practitioners interested in the field of epigenetics. They offer conferences, resources, and publications.

3. The Babraham Institute

- A leading research institute focusing on the molecular mechanisms underlying normal cellular processes and their dysfunction in diseases. Their research on epigenetics is internationally recognized.

For those interested in learning more about epigenetics and human longevity, the above resources provide a roadmap to further exploration. While the field is complex, the potential it holds for our understanding of human biology, health, disease, and longevity is boundless.